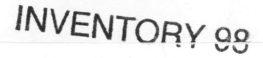

MAN
TO MAN

MAN TO MAN

When the Woman You Love Has Breast Cancer

Andy Murcia and Bob Stewart

ST. MARTIN'S PRESS · New York

Design by Joan Jacobus

Library of Congress Cataloging-in-Publication Data

Murcia, Andy.
    Man to man.

    1. Breast—Cancer—Patients—Family relationships.
2. Married people. I. Stewart, Bob. II. Title.
RC280.B8M84 1989   616.99'449   88-30563
ISBN 0-312-02605-6

First Edition
10 9 8 7 6 5 4 3 2 1

To Ann and Martha—
  you are the love of our lives.

And to all the other women and their families and
  friends—this book is dedicated to all of you.

Contents

Foreword

Breast cancer will affect one in ten American women. Although it is the most common form of cancer among women, certainly none of them—or the men in their lives—is ever prepared for such a diagnosis.

Andy Murcia and Bob Stewart readily admit they were paralyzed with panic when they learned in the same week that their wives had breast cancer. Here were two tough men—Andy is a former Chicago policeman and Bob a San Antonio newspaper reporter—stunned over the possibility of losing their wives, actress Ann Jillian and homemaker Martha Stewart. Nothing in their earlier years could compare with either the physical or psychological struggles that stretched over months of therapy before Ann and Martha returned to good health.

Fortunately, these two friends reached out to each other. Through numerous phone calls from California to Texas, Andy and Bob shared their worst fears. They cried, prayed, and laughed together; one or the other usually had a tip on what was working right then to help Ann or Martha through an especially difficult phase of treatment. Once long-term survival for their wives seemed probable, Andy and Bob decided to write a book that would provide the solace and advice they had not had to aid other men faced with similar ordeals.

In *Man to Man,* they discuss virtually all aspects of their experiences, from getting a second medical opinion and gaining knowledge about the disease to coping with side effects of chemotherapy and encouraging their wives to do post-surgical exercises. They offer dozens of commonsense recommendations for setting realistic goals during therapy, overcoming emotional logjams, and enjoying intimacies while recovering from cancer.

The authors emphasize that a combination of faith, hope, and love are essential for any man to endure the battle of breast cancer with his wife. "You will need faith in today's modern medical science, you will need hope to keep your spirits high, and you will need love for everything," they write.

Andy and Bob concede that there is tremendous comfort in some old clichés. Stopping to smell the roses, taking one day at a time, understanding that money cannot buy happiness, *and* appreciating that when you have your health you have everything all took on new meanings for both couples. They talk about crying, alone and with their wives, but they also stress the value of laughter. "A sense of humor can be one of your most important assets in the battle against cancer," they say, going on to cite examples of how good humor helped in even the bleakest of situations.

Man to Man is a long-overdue book that should prove invaluable to any man whose wife or other loved one is confronted with breast cancer. While Andy and Bob convey solid medical information on diagnosis and treatment options, readers undoubtedly will appreciate most their hints on dealing with the depression that see-saws through any serious illness and suggestions for helping their wives face life without breasts.

This is an extraordinary book, poignantly written from the hearts of two men who, with their special wives, have learned to cherish life after cancer.

Charles A. LeMaistre, M.D.
President
The University of Texas M. D. Anderson Cancer Center

Prologue

Two men. Friends. Each facing the same problems. Fearful, often confused. Not knowing where to turn during those emotional early days, they reached out across half a continent to help each other.

Man to man, they shared their fears, their problems, their secret thoughts. They helped each other make decisions, exchanged newfound knowledge, and provided emotional support.

These were new, uncharted seas for them, and they wished desperately for some type of map to guide them through the problems that lay ahead in their wives' battle with breast cancer.

Two women. The actress and the housewife. Friends. Each facing the same problem, yet each forced to undergo different treatment. Fearful, often confused, they turned to their husbands for primary support in a battle fo

It was the most important role thos
played. They were ill-prepared, but they toug
new strength through faith, hope, and love a
only their wives but also each other to ove
challenge.

We know, because we are those men. When our wives were stricken, we would have given anything for cohesive information we could have used to help them cope. We needed knowledge, and we needed it fast. And we needed a psychological guide for both us and our wives.

We believe this book answers many important questions we had to wrestle with—and find answers for—while traveling the rocky road to our wives' survival. Those answers were often difficult to come by and we learned some of them the hard way: through trial and error.

We have also found that there is an invaluable network of shared experiences that will help you cope. But when you deal with cancer, no two cases are alike. Each couple must seek its own solutions, as we did, while freely drawing on the shared experience of others, as we did.

We hope our experiences will ease your burden, smooth your path, and minimize your own trial and error. We know that if you've ever wanted to help anyone in your life, it is right now. We believe our solutions will help both you and your wife deal with a difficult disease. They will also help a mother or father or brother or sister or any relative or friend joining you in this battle.

And, finally, as we did for each other, we hope to reach out from these pages and give you support, man to man.

Andy Murcia
Bob Stewart

MAN
TO MAN

1

You're Never Prepared

Bob: I was scared. Gut-wrenching, numbingly scared. I had faced problems before, but nothing like this.

I can't say exactly why I reached out to Andy that morning. I knew he was a sensitive, caring person, but that wasn't it. Maybe I was looking for the cop in him—the tough, no-nonsense dependability he developed while working vice in a city as tough as Chicago.

Perhaps it was something as simple as friendship. Ours is unique. Andy is a sincere, fast-talking product of Brooklyn who married entertainer Ann Jillian. Me? I'm a tall, small-town South Texan married to a woman content to be a housewife.

I didn't have time to think about it then. Things happened so fast that I didn't telephone until after the biopsy and Martha's first chemotherapy treatment.

"Andy, Martha's got breast cancer," I said.

"How bad?"

"Bad enough the doctors can't remove it. It's too big. They have to try to shrink it before they can perform surgery," I said. "It's in her breast and lymph nodes."

"How did you spot it?" he asked.

1

"She's been monitoring it for nearly nine months and the doc said everything was all right until now," I explained.

I'll always wonder if indecision on my part put Martha's life in greater jeopardy. After the doctors discovered fibrocystic growths, we debated the need for a biopsy.

"Unless we actually look, we can't be one hundred percent sure there is no cancer there," the doctor told us. All the indicators had pointed to fibrocystic disease (a benign condition of liquid-filled cysts), which appeared smooth and rounded on her original mammogram more than a year before. A mammogram performed only a few weeks before the cancer turned her breast red and angry had confirmed only the presence of fibrocystic cysts. It is very rare for a mammogram to miss the presence of cancer and we later learned that the cancer had been hiding behind interconnected fibrocystic cysts and muscle. Martha was reluctant to face the knife. She had had major surgery three times before. None of them had been for cancer, but they had been enough to make her dread more surgery. After talking to several doctors, she decided to have the liquid cysts drained by needle and monitored.

"Aspiration won't solve the problem a hundred percent," I argued of the needle technique that emptied the cysts and eased the painful condition. Aspiration could not tell us if cancer was lurking behind a healthy muscle or in the fibrocystic cyst. Nor would a needle biopsy. What if it missed the cancer? The only one hundred percent solution was an examination of the site and removal of the cysts through surgery. But I didn't press the point in my talks with Martha because I, too, didn't want her to have still another general anesthesia.

Months of success lulled us into complacency. Then one day the doctor couldn't get the needle into one of the lumps in Martha's left breast. For the second time in a year he wanted a biopsy, but we waited. After all, a mammogram just a week earlier had shown no sign of a malignant tumor. In the next few weeks her breast grew bruised, swollen, and red.

Finally we had no choice but biopsy. When Martha's doctor came into the waiting room, his first words were: "It's a wildly growing carcinoma."

He might as well have told me she was dead. The three of us—my son, daughter, and I—tried to console each other. The tumultuous waiting room was filled with nearly twenty weeping friends and relatives.

The doctor stepped forward and hugged me, "I'm sorry," he said, so frustrated he was nearly shouting. "You know I would have done something if I could."

I felt sorry for both of us.

The cancer was so large he was fearful of removing it. He whittled away a portion, but decided additional surgery might cause it to spread further. Martha would receive chemotherapy and radiation with the goal of reducing the tumor to a manageable size for surgery. Survival was estimated at less than fifty percent.

The uncertainty of Martha's future filled me with stone-cold fear. Mingled with it was an aching remorse: I should have insisted that she have the biopsy when the lump was first discovered. Failing that, I should have insisted on a biopsy when the tumor couldn't be aspirated just a few weeks before.

Martha and I talked about it. In fact, we talked about little else. In times of stress you turn to your best friend, but mine was in a hospital bed devastated by chemotherapy, terrified beyond description; perhaps that's why I called Andy.

"Bob," Andy hesitated, after I told him what had happened. Then the words rushed out:

"Ann has a lump, and I don't know what to do."

"I do," I told him. "Get her to a doctor and get her there fast. If he says biopsy, then get one. I wish I had—with all my heart."

Now it was two very scared men who hung up the telephone.

———

Andy: Because she didn't want to worry me, Ann and her doctors had quietly monitored the lump for several months. I had learned about it only a few days before Bob called.

Another trip to the doctor confirmed our fears. I couldn't

have been more staggered than if someone had struck me in the belly with a sledgehammer.

I knew that if anyone could understand how I now felt, it would be Bob. Ours has been a long-distance friendship of frequent letters and telephone calls and infrequent visits when he and Martha were in California on business or when Ann and I went to San Antonio for personal appearances.

Bob is one of those tall Texans with a Southwestern drawl that makes two words out of one. He's a bit on the serious side and I have to loosen him up from time to time. I've often told him that if I had to go into a dark alley, I'd want him at my back. This was the darkest alley I'd been down.

By the time I got back in touch with Bob, Ann and I knew what we had to do.

"Not only does Ann have cancer, but she has it in both breasts," I told him. "The doctors want to take both of them."

By his silence, I could tell that Bob was stunned. Like me he's seldom at a loss for words. But I had had trouble finding the right words for him just a few days ago.

"What do they say about her chances?" Bob said.

"That's the good news. They think she'll be all right. It's contained, and in those cases they say survival odds are over ninety percent."

"Then get her in there and get it done. Fast," he urged.

Bob sounded so positive—so sure that immediate action should be taken. "I will," I said.

"How are you doing?" he asked.

"I'll be okay, Bob, but I just don't know what to do for her. When the life of the person you love more than anyone else is being threatened, it's the most helpless feeling in the world."

"I know," he said. "If it were some guy with a knife or a gun or something like that, you could step in between. You'd have something to fight. That wouldn't be any problem. You'd take on anything, but this . . ." he paused. "It's the most helpless feeling in the world. Martha has always said that when you have your health, you have everything."

"Bob, if I could take everything we have and give it to

someone and they could guarantee Ann wouldn't have this, I'd do it, gladly. I'd live in poverty," I said.

Later I would learn that fear and anger, even bargaining, were all part of the process of dealing with life-threatening illness. I was so scared. I had already lost my mother and sister to cancer.

"Ann's scared," I said before admitting, "Hell, I'm scared, too."

"Martha and I were scared, too, but we learned to get it done, and the sooner the better," he said. "After all, you want Annie. You're not concerned about Ann Jillian the television star. And we've both fooled around with breasts enough to last the rest of our lives. What do we need them for, when we can have our wives?"

"You're right," I agreed. "The important thing is saving her life. What do Ann and I need breasts for when we have each other?"

"That's the way I see it," Bob answered.

It was the obvious, calming, commonsense approach to the dilemma, which we would both cling to like drowning men clutching a stick. And it helped to have a friend state the obvious and shore up my floundering common sense.

These were conversations that would be repeated many times, in many forms, during the next two years. There would be shared tears and prayers and fears and eventually joy as Ann and Martha reclaimed their roles in life.

The conversations were good for both of us. By reaching out man to man, each of us realized that there was another person in this world who understood exactly how he felt.

No matter what hour a call came or how painful the topic, when each of us hung up the phone, we were refreshed, ready to resume the battle.

These conversations helped us cut through the confusion of the moment. We know there is confusion. Like every other person who faces this disease with a loved one, we were forced to take a crash course on its effects and cures. We made mistakes; sometimes we waited too long to act, and other times we were too hasty. Sometimes we felt like we made every mistake in the book. We would like to help you lay out your own blueprint of battle and get you started on the road to treatment with a commonsense approach that includes examples based on our own experiences. Most of all, we want you to realize that there is life during and after cancer.

We understand how you feel upon learning that a woman you love has breast cancer. You are facing one of life's most dramatic challenges. We know this is true, because we have faced the same challenge.

We have felt fearful, angry, resentful, depressed, and hopeful—some days, all at the same time.

There was no way in the world we could have been prepared for what was about to happen when the doctors told Ann and Martha that they had breast cancer.

Although cancer is one of the top three potential killers in this country—statistics for women alone show that one out of every ten will get breast cancer—you actually give it little thought, except for the occasional instance when it strikes a friend or when a news story sparks interest. To say you are unprepared is an understatement. Even Andy, who had already lost a mother and sister to cancer, was unprepared for the emotional tumult that followed Ann's diagnosis.

But there is help and hope today for a disease whose diagnosis was once considered an automatic death sentence, thanks to:

- Early detection through self-examination and mammographies
- Heightened public awareness brought about by some celebrities and public figures who do not hesitate to tell their story
- A growing interest in health by both men and women
- A dramatic cut in the time it takes for the results of laboratory research to become available to doctors and the public

- Aggressive methods of treatment through surgery, chemo-therapy, and radiation that sustain life longer
- Follow-up care through medical checkups, stress control, diet, and exercise

If the cancer has not spread beyond its primary site (contained), a woman is given better than a ninety percent chance to survive. And modern treatment has so extended lives that it is not uncommon for a woman to have had the disease and to return to her normal routine. There is a growing legion of former cancer patients, all members of an unofficial "sisterhood," a label Ann used in a *People* magazine interview.

But, as you stand there, knees knocking and fear ripping your heart out when you first hear the diagnosis, you need a good dose of common sense and reassurance, and a game plan to get treatment started. A man who has just heard the news is filled with thousands of questions and buffeted by ten thousand emotions.

Will she die? Am I reacting properly? How honest should I be? How do I make an intelligent decision? How will I feel the first time I see my wife without a breast? Will she misread my fears and attentions as meaning that death is imminent? How do I know to trust this particular doctor? Should I cry in front of her? Should I talk privately with the doctor? Should I let her know that I'm scared, too? Is cancer contagious?

The questions tumble out unendingly. Chances are that's why you are reading this book. No one can claim to have all the answers, but we do have the solutions we worked out when facing the above questions, and dozens of others. And we believe these answers will give you and your wife a chance to grasp and cope with the situation and proceed with some semblance of order.

What should you do first? You do two things that are purely emotional. First, we challenge you to put yourself into her shoes. Everyone fears illness and its attendant treatment, especially if it means surgery or long days of recovery. But can you understand her emotional state? At best this will be difficult. Obviously a man does not place the same sexual identity on his breasts a woman does; obviously it will be difficult to project himself into her situation because he cannot suffer the exact loss. But consider: How would you feel if you were forced to face the possibility of losing a portion of your sexuality? You may find it easier to understand her fear of death than to relate to a loss that can sap her self-confidence, especially in a society that places such an emphasis on breasts.

Second, if you haven't already, you may have to grow up. Maturity should be a never-ending process and we found ourselves learning new depths of maturity almost daily. Bob discovered a leaflet entitled "Steps to Maturity" during one of Martha's early hospital stays. We believe it to be a good guide and offer it as an aid in coping with your present difficulties. You may consider copying it and putting it on the mirror in your bathroom. It gives us a boost each time we feel weak.

STEPS TO MATURITY

Maturity is the ability to handle frustration, control anger, and settle differences without violence or destruction.

Maturity is patience. It is the willingness to postpone gratification, to pass up the immediate pleasure or profit in favor of the long-term gain.

Maturity is perseverance, sweating out a project or a situation in spite of opposition and discouraging setbacks.

Maturity is unselfishness, responding to the needs of others.

Maturity is the capacity to face unpleasantness and disappointment without becoming bitter.

Maturity is the gift of remaining calm in the face of chaos. This means peace, not only for ourselves, but for those with whom we live and for those whose lives touch ours.

Maturity is the ability to disagree without being disagreeable.

Maturity is humility. A mature person is able to say, "I was wrong." He is also able to say, "I am sorry." And when he is proven right he does not have to say, "I told you so."

Maturity is the ability to make a decision, to act on that decision, and to accept full responsibility for the outcome.

Maturity means dependability, integrity, keeping one's word. The immature have excuses for everything. They are the chronically tardy, the no-shows, the gutless wonders who fold in the crisis. Their lives are a maze of broken promises, unfinished business, and former friends.

Maturity is the ability to live in peace with that which we cannot change.

—Anonymous

While men may not suffer the physical pain and agony of surgery, they often suffer a similar mental anguish—rooted in fear of the unknown—as their loved ones.

Within the first few days, you will be called on to make life-or-death decisions that will tax your physical and mental capacities. You must face the possibility of death (How do I find out what those statistics mean?) while launching the battle for survival by securing second and even third opinions (How do I do that?).

Knowledge is power in this battle. (But how do you become educated?) We have pieced together a picture of our battles so that you won't have to search frantically through dozens of brochures on chemotherapy, surgery, and radiation or wade through highly technical clinical explanations, which often are confusing.

You need a game plan that moves logically from diagnosis to second opinion to medical treatment to emotional sustenance.

Participation is the key. As you amass knowledge, you will be better prepared to handle family needs, protect your wife from horror stories told by well-meaning friends and relatives, stand by her side during medical treatment, shore up her often fragile mental state, and ease her return to the world. Knowledge will also help erase fear.

Exercise, diet, and a positive self-image will follow initial victories as you look to the future.

"Now abideth faith, hope, and love," Saint Paul writes in the thirteenth chapter of First Corinthians. "And the greatest of these is love."

You will need faith in today's modern medical science, you will need hope to keep your spirits high, and you will need love for everything.

You have been plunged into a world where faith and hope are the watchdogs of sanity and health; and love is what keeps them vigilant. Medical experts have told us many times that the majority of women who successfully negotiate these treacherous waters are the ones with the strongest support system composed of husbands, family, and friends who share faith, hope, and love. When you combine this with the wonderful professionals of the medical team, who compose the first line of defense, then you have a powerful positive force for healing.

And finally, there will be changes—in both you and your wife—but we believe these changes can be positive forces to draw you closer together. From the moment we learned that our wives had breast cancer our lives changed forever.

It's up to you to determine how your life will be changed. Some couples have responded to the challenge by drawing closer together, their lives more intertwined than ever before. Some couples have grown apart, or even divorced, on the rare occasions when the burden became too heavy. We hope your burden never becomes that heavy. None of us is truly prepared for the sacrifices and struggles that come with the territory. We certainly weren't prepared. We expected our lives to remain as happy as the night we all finally met in 1981.

Bob: Ann Jillian had just charmed the growl right out of the wolf pack. Standing with her arms stretched to the ceiling, a microphone dangling from one hand, she gracefully acknowledged the applause of the nation's television editors as it bounced off the walls of a small banquet room in the Beverly Hills Hotel.

Ann had created a sensation the year before when ABC-TV premiered the television sitcom, "It's a Living." Although she'd been performing since childhood, it was the first time television columnists and editors had discovered her. She was showcased as Cassie Cranston, a wise-cracking, brassy blonde. The characterization stole the show and captured the hearts of the cynical critics who had gathered for the annual screening of upcoming television series slated to air that fall.

But it wasn't only Cassie who sparkled. Ann's effervescent personality captivated the crowd. She was fresh, outgoing and friendly, but still a professional who knew how to handle herself. A biography prepared by the network pointed out that her credits were mostly television and stage, although she had appeared in such movies as Babes in Toyland *for Walt Disney (who changed her Lithuanian name from Ann Jura Nauseda to Ann Jillian) and* Gypsy. *(Ann played the role of Dainty June, Gypsy's younger sister.) Many of the critics had just seen her perform in the original Broadway cast of* Sugar Babies, *the highly acclaimed Mickey Rooney/Ann Miller Broadway show that resurrected vaudeville.*

Traditionally, the networks trot out stars for interview sessions after screenings. Like the rest of the writers there, I was intrigued by the character of Cassie, a savvy waitress who seemed to have spunk and substance—along with a heart of gold. But something happened during that interview that made me more interested in the actress than the character she played.

The interview had been centering on Cassie, the sex symbol. Everyone was curious about the platinum-blond Dutch-boy–cut hairstyle Ann wore as Cassie, and which has since become her trademark. Questions were asked about the public perception of Cassie, the impact of the character as a role model for children, and the possibility of Cassie becoming a breakout character from the show.

Finally a reporter said:

"You've been around this industry for years and now it appears you're getting your first big break and big money. How has it affected you? What things have you been able to do now that you've always wanted to do?"

Ann didn't hesitate. "I was able to buy a house for my parents. For years they devoted themselves to my career. I didn't even realize we were poor until I had grown up. The biggest payoff of all is not in having money, but in being able to spend it on them."

She smiled and continued, "But believe it or not, I couldn't convince my folks that I was doing well until they read about me in a Lithuanian newspaper."

That drew a laugh from the newspaper crowd, who could appreciate the irony of a small, foreign-language publication meaning more to her parents than papers representing millions in circulation.

Then the questions returned to Ann Jillian, the glamorous star. I was fascinated. Here was a woman who contradicted the stereotype. All she had to do was give the critics a few brassy Cassie lines, bat her eyelashes, and project the bad-girl image. Instead, she came across as a wholesome, all-American girl, more interested in family than fame, and eager to share what she had earned with her loved ones. She was a fresh voice in the "me" generation.

When the session ended, I went straight to Joe Maggio, an ABC-TV publicist.

"Joe, when I get home, I want a phoner with Ann Jillian," I said, referring to a telephone interview.

"Let's do it now," Joe suggested.

"I'd rather wait. Just tell her I want to talk to her about her family."

"Her family?" Joe laughed.

A month later when Ann telephoned the newspaper where I wrote a daily television column, she sounded incredulous. *"You really want to talk about my parents?"*

"Yes," I replied.

The actress who played the alluring Cassie is a first-generation American. Her parents are naturalized citizens who came to America from Lithuania, fleeing the Russian advance during the closing days of World War II.

After leaving a life of privilege, her father and mother took whatever jobs they could to support their family in Cambridge, Massachusetts, where Ann was born. Her mother noticed Ann's talent as a child and insisted the family move to Hollywood to give her every opportunity.

By the time the interview was over, I knew what I'd use for my lead, and it appeared the next week as a cover story in the Sunday television guide.

"Ann Jillian is a beautiful example of the American dream," I wrote and went on to tell her story.

A few weeks later I received the first of many notes from Ann and her husband, Andy Murcia.

"I cried when I read the story," Ann wrote.

She followed up with a telephone call to tell me that the story had been framed and put in the hallway entrance of their Sherman Oaks home.

From this exchange began a tentative friendship that developed into note writing and an occasional telephone call. But despite our growing relationship, none of us had ever met.

That didn't happen until the night of Ann's performance.

It was also a special time for me. I was reared in the dusty small towns of South Texas. As a youngster—like the majority *of the kids—I spent a few days each summer pulling cotton to earn spending money. The biggest event in these little havens of security was Friday night football or a band concert or high school play. And then, there was the motion picture theater where for nine cents you could see a years-old movie. I read every book I could find and especially loved the old silver-screen magazines with their fanciful stories about the stars.*

I had made a pledge during my youth that I would one day meet these people. And now, I was there; a part of my life's dream fulfilled. It was a special moment.

During the performance, I kept telling Martha, my very bemused wife, to expect anything when Ann and I first met.

"Oh sure, she's going to grab you and kiss you," Martha teased.

"She might," I replied, now a little embarrassed for even bringing it up. Martha had had no contact with Ann or Andy, and I wanted her to like them as much as I did.

"I'll see if I can control myself," Martha continued to tease. I often amused her because of my unabashed interest in the entertainment industry. She was reared around show business. Her mother, Lillian Murphy, was a singer who toured with stage shows as a teenager, and her grandmother, Mattie Williams, was seamstress for the show. Later her mother would be a nightclub performer and Martha would spend most of her youth living with her grandmother. Other members of her family traveled the carnival circuit; so, when Martha had a birthday as a little girl in Dallas, she had clowns and dancers and vaudeville acts to entertain her guests. Her grandmother could spin some great stories, having known such diverse individuals as entertainer Al Jolson and outlaws Bonnie Parker and Clyde Barrow.

As the evening's entertainment ended that night in Hollywood, Ann began to work the crowd, visiting with the columnists, most of whom she knew or had talked to on the telephone. "I sure enjoyed your show," I told her as she came up.

We discussed the show and she told me it was composed

largely of songs she used in Las Vegas. We hit a lull in the conversation.

"Are you having a good time?" she asked politely.

"Yes, meeting you has been one of the highlights of the trip," I replied.

"Oh! Where are you from? What's your name?" she asked as she looked at my name tag for the first time.

"Bob Stewart," she said before doing a double take. "You're Bob Stewart."

Before I knew it, she did *grab me and hug me, jumping up and down.*

Me? I was laughing.

Martha? She was laughing and taking pictures. Ann saw her and exclaimed, "I'll give you something to take a picture of" and planted a kiss on my cheek before signaling across the room,

"Andy, here's Bob Stewart."

I looked up to see a bear of a man bounding across the room, a big grin on his face. Andy Murcia grabbed my hand and started pumping it. When everything settled down, I introduced them to Martha.

Andy explained that my stories had struck a responsive chord with him and Ann because they, too, had pictured her as the All-American girl-next-door.

"We see her as America's sweetheart," said Andy. "It's a clean and attractive image. It's Ann, as opposed to the 'sex bomb' tag the press puts on her."

It was a wonderful, warm evening that cemented what was to become a deep and lasting friendship. Life was sweet for all of us that night. Little did we know the trials and tribulations we would soon share.

2

The Discovery

Andy: I can read faces pretty darn well. I spent eighteen years working as a cop in Chicago, and if a cop could not read the face of a guy coming at him, he was a good candidate for getting hurt on the job.

When the doctor walked into his office where Ann and I were awaiting test results, I knew we were both candidates for getting hurt. I could tell that the news was bad; I just didn't know how bad. It didn't take long to find out. By the time he got to the part about Ann needing a double mastectomy and that it wasn't just his opinion, but that of the radiologist, I could feel my chest constrict. Then I was filled with anger. Then I was worried about Ann. How was she taking it? I looked at her. She was calm, angry in a silent way. And after eight years of marriage, I could read her face, too; and there was no fear, only anger.

I was mad enough for both of us. I jumped to my feet, towering over the doctor who remained seated.

"What the hell do we do now?" I demanded. "How come it took you guys so long to tell what the hell it is?"

By now I'm yelling, all two hundred-plus pounds quivering with rage.

"Well, I think you're wrong, Doc," I shouted as I turned to Ann.

It was nothing but pure bluster, because in my heart of hearts, deep down inside I was thinking:

Oh, God, I've lost her.

But there was no way in the world I would have let Ann know what I was thinking at that exact moment.

"Come on, babe, let's get out of here. We'll get another opinion and more if we need them."

I felt as if my anger, my yelling, my refusing to believe what the doctor had told us, would make it all go away. Of course it didn't, but that was my reaction.

I also thought that as a good husband I could protect Ann from the truth a little while longer if she saw that I did not believe it. It was a desperate attempt to comfort her. I couldn't help but wonder what her poor mind was going through.

I was later to discover that disbelieving is a normal first reaction and that anger at the medical folks is a close second.

I was scared to death. My knees got weak like someone had delivered a Sunday punch right on the jaw and I was about to go down.

In a few minutes, I had it under control. I felt sorry for Ann. I even felt sorry for the doc who was just sitting there wringing his hands, with tears starting to form in his eyes.

"What I told you I would tell my own sister, or wife, if I had one," he continued calmly. "And I respect your right to get other opinions if you desire them. But I must advise you: Do not wait too long. Get the other opinions fast and let's get on with saving Ann's life."

That seemed to settle me down. It was obvious he was not trying to hurt us. He had deep, good feelings for us. He was on our side and wanted only to save Ann's life.

It was a long ride home that afternoon. I wanted to get caught up on what had been happening, so I questioned her. I had just learned that she and my sister, Joanie, had been watching a small, pea-sized "pimple" on the top of her left breast. That's what I'd just found out about when I talked to Bob.

She had had a mammogram of both breasts and the doctors had been watching her. The first doctor wanted a biopsy; then Ann went to an internist for a second opinion.

"She told me that we'd watch it," Ann said rather ruefully as we drove home. "I finally found a doctor to tell me what I wanted to hear," she explained.

Several months after seeing the internist, the bras in her Las Vegas costumes began hurting her. She calls them "rawhide bras" because they "head 'em up and move 'em out."

"When I got home and was doing my exercises, I decided I'd better get this checked," she continued. "I kept pulling my knee up and it kept touching my right breast and whenever it did the breast felt funny.

"I can't really describe how it feels, Andy, except to say that it feels like my breast is full of old foam rubber," she said.

To my chagrin, I hadn't noticed anything.

We had already decided to get a second opinion following that day's doctor's visit, and a plan was forming in my mind as I drove home to make sure she got the best second opinion possible.

"Is there anything else I don't know?" I asked her, feeling a little guilty because the question made me sound more like a policeman than a husband. What she couldn't see was the fear and love in my heart.

"No," she said quietly. She stopped talking. I felt like I understood and we rode home in silence.

We passed many familiar landmarks along the way, some of them soundstages and auditoriums where Ann had tasted sweet success. One was a soundstage where that very afternoon she would be recording a song for *Alice in Wonderland*. At that moment, success, money, fame, fortune—even breasts—were not important. All I wanted was for her to live. That's all I have ever wanted since that day. It's the first thing I ask for in my prayers. I say,

"Dear God, keep cancer away from her and let her die an old doll of at least ninety years."

Even though there has been a diagnosis of cancer, *all is not lost.*

While it's true that this expression is a cliché, you've probably never understood until now the phrase's rich, emotional textures. Unfortunately, in a very short time you will come to understand a lot of clichés: You will yearn to stop and smell the roses; you will understand why money cannot buy happiness; you will learn to live one day at a time; you will be touched by the knowledge that if you have your health you have everything; you know, all too well, that time will tell. Any cliché you've mouthed all your life now settles into the very fiber of your being to become a slogan at one time or another that not only you, but also doctors and nurses, use to sustain hope in a desperate physical and mental battle.

All of us understand that death is inevitable. We know we can't escape it. We learn to live with it by dismissing it from the present. Except for tragic circumstances, death is something that happens to the elderly; so, for the most part, it is something in our far distant future. But the word "cancer" has the ability to make the future present, and death a reality. When cancer enters your life, even the most mundane plans involving the future take on new meaning.

For the first time you realize that a person must savor the small moments of life. Now, you regret all the times you let those fleeting moments go by—the missed birthdays, the un-whispered "I love yous," the postponed weekend trips—everything you now fear you ever missed comes crashing down on you. Suddenly it seems as if there is not enough time.

Think! If you feel all of this, how does *she* feel? If you are scared and in an emotional whirlwind, how much more terrifying must it be for the one who actually has the life-threatening disease?

The two of you will feel emotions not unlike those experienced at the death of a loved one. Unfortunately you do not have the time for a long period of adjustment. You must act swiftly to ensure the best medical treatment and that includes working your way through this emotional jungle. A combination of emotions will assail you, sometimes singularly, sometimes all at once. Fear is the predominate emotion and it's okay to be fearful. It's a natural state; just don't let it paralyze you.

Psychologists have discovered a basic pattern in which shock and disbelief are the first reactions after fear. Most women do not even feel the slightest illness at diagnosis, so it is easy to believe that the doctor could be wrong. Most women receive an evaluation because they felt a lump—something that just doesn't feel right—not pain or fever or any of the traditional signposts of illness.

Sometimes disbelief is followed by denial—a particularly dangerous stage because some people go through a series of second opinions until they find one they like.

Denial is dangerous.

Bob: On one occasion, Martha turned to me and for one brief moment tried to deny the obvious.

"I think I'll just not have the surgery. It'd probably be okay," she said during the long months of radiation and chemotherapy. "If it weren't for you and the children, I'd just leave it alone and take my chances. I'm living on borrowed time anyway."

It was a desperate attempt to escape the reality of the situation by deciding that everything would be okay if you just ignored it.

Anger ("Why me?" she asks, "Why her?" you ask) or blame ("I deserve this") or bargaining (God, you do this for me and I'll do some good deed in your name) are the next emotional logjams. Depression and anxiety settle in, sometimes immobilizing the patient.

Be particularly careful of blame. In some cases, the cancer patient develops the attitude that cancer is her just reward; her life has not been good enough to warrant good health. Remove those doubts; it is your job to give her reassurance.

Recognize all these emotions for what they are—especially anger, which sometimes you will direct at one another—and do not let them interfere with your relationship. You need each other now more than ever.

Often tension will be more intense at the time of diagnosis or at the time you begin treatment (surgery, chemotherapy, or radiation). Stress will also intensify when awaiting test results (this is an especially difficult time) or when trying to make a decision concerning treatment. Understanding your emotional state and taking swift action not only assures immediate medical attention, but also helps ease stress.

And then, finally, comes acceptance; not of death, but of the reality of the situation. Don't confuse this with "resignation." Acceptance doesn't mean you have accepted defeat or death. With acceptance comes the courage to continue the battle.

You are in the fight of your life with your sole aim being to defeat the disease. You will weep, you will be angry, you will rage at the fates, but you will come to grips with the problem, *swiftly,* and take an active role in the battle. Work your way through these emotions and bring yourself under control as soon as possible so you can forge ahead aggressively. You are probably in for a long struggle, so don't expect any quick, easy solutions. Just hang in there.

Bob: It seemed almost impossible to control the raging anguish that began when Martha called from the doctor's office.

Medical problems were nothing new to us. In the twenty-six years we've been married, she has had a kidney removed, the other repaired, and peritonitis from a perforated colon that eventually led to a colon resection. These were all congenital problems, unrelated to cancer, a disease unknown among the women of Martha's family.

Adversity was nothing new. There were even times when

we weren't sure she would survive, but a tenacious spirit always asserted itself and she soon regained her place in life.

This time it was different. A fear I had never known coursed through me as I rushed to meet her at home. The doctor had told me in no uncertain terms that he believed—no, knew!—that it was cancer, based on his long years of experience.

Shaken to the core, Martha had called from the doctor's office. I hadn't gone with her that day, because we thought it was going to be just another routine visit.

"Doctor, I know Martha is standing there, so please answer 'yes' or 'no' or 'I think so,' so she won't be any more scared than she already is," I said when I got on the telephone.

"Do you think it is cancer?" I asked.

"Yes, sir," was his even-voiced reply.

"I know you need a biopsy to be absolutely sure, but your experience doesn't leave any doubt, does it?" I continued.

"No, sir," he said.

"Do you think it's cancer because of what your hands tell you when you examine her breast?" I asked.

"Yes, sir. And my eyes," he added.

"Does it look real bad?"

"I think so," he said.

"Then we need to get something done immediately?" It was more of a statement than a question.

"As soon as possible, like this Monday," he said.

"Is she emotionally stable enough to drive?"

"I think so," the doctor replied.

"Then let me talk to her, please."

"Martha," I began, "go home and I'll be right there. We'll decide what to do," I said, trying to sound as reassuring and confident as possible, although my heart pounded in my chest and my emotions screamed for release.

"Bob, I'm scared," she said.

"It'll be okay. Your doctor is one of the best surgeons in the business," I told her.

I hung up and went straight to the newspaper's executive editor.

"The doctors believe Martha has cancer." My voice broke and tears began to ease down my cheeks.

"I'm sorry. Go home and take care of your wife. We'll work everything out here. Right now, she should be your first concern. Let me know what happens," he said, giving immediate support.

"I'll let you know as soon as we find out what we're going to do," I called back as I headed out the door.

This discovery came after more than a year of monitoring fibrocystic disease in both of Martha's breasts. Because we had tried to be so careful, the doctor's words were all the more numbing.

My thoughts whizzed through the past year. When the lumps were discovered, every doctor had told us that the only way to be a hundred percent certain they were not malignant was to perform a biopsy. Martha feared more surgery and since the rounded, even-edged X rays had indicated we were dealing with fibrocystic disease—which is usually noncancerous—it was decided to use a needle and drain the liquid-filled lumps instead of going ahead with the surgical procedure. This had been done twice previously; only this time the lumps didn't drain.

It was a difficult session. Try as he could, the surgeon couldn't get the needle into one of the lumps to drain it. He recommended going ahead with the biopsy, but Martha declined; the X rays taken just a few weeks before had indicated no sign of cancer. It was decided to wait. Within six weeks her left breast was slightly swollen and an angry red color. We didn't think anything about it. We suspected that it was bruised from the session with the needle when the cyst couldn't be drained. So, when Martha left for the doctor that morning, we weren't overly concerned about the outcome. None of us had any idea that a cancer was present since the mammogram—which normally catches even the smallest of tumors—was clear and the doctor's clinical examination did not reveal it. The term "one hundred percent" kept echoing in my mind. Only a biopsy would have revealed what until now had been a hidden cancer. One second-opinion doctor would later estimate she had had it for a number of years.

As I pulled into the driveway, I put on a poker face—I knew I couldn't let her see how this news had affected me. I mustered all my courage as I walked across the lawn, but when I took her in my arms, I cried like a baby. We held each other tight, unable to completely comfort each other, both of us weeping with deep racking sobs. Months later she told me that she thought she was dead for sure because of my reaction.

It was the better part of an hour before we regained our composure, bleakly looked at each other, and began the long journey to survival.

We had to get second opinions immediately and make hospital reservations for Martha. The surgeon was especially urgent. He wanted the biopsy done Monday if at all possible. It was late Friday afternoon and we had only scant hours before doctors' offices and hospitals shut down for the weekend.

3

The Many Faces of Fear

"We have nothing to fear but fear itself." —Franklin Delano Roosevelt

Cancer is an emotionally charged word: You can't be neutral about it. Because cancer has become synonymous with life-threatening, no other disease provokes such dread. Like us, you have probably heard so many horror stories about cancer that your first reaction is fear: fear of the unknown; fear of suffering; fear of death.

That fear is the reason many women delay getting lumps checked. Fear can cost lives, so we challenge you to bring this emotion under control. If you are immobilized and don't know which way to turn, it's that old bogeyman, fear.

FDR, while leading this country out of the Great Depression and through a world war, undoubtedly knew fear. Although paralyzed from an adult bout with polio, he mastered the fear that accompanied that terrible disease and rose to great heights. His famous and grand statement about fearing fear itself has become an American watchword.

Cancer can be a killer; but not always. Because it has become so prevalent, everyone knows someone who has died from it. But chances are they also know someone who is still alive years after a doctor told the patient she had less than six months to live. And we've never met a doctor who doesn't delight in being wrong! The problem is that these success stories slip from the mind as time goes by, seldom to resurface, while our reservoir of fear is constantly being replenished with each new death.

Now that cancer has been diagnosed, two considerations—so closely interwoven that they are almost impossible to separate—will doubtlessly begin to dominate your thoughts: your wife's statistical chances for survival and the possibility of her death. So, let's discuss both of these concerns right away and get on with the battle.

AVOID THE NUMBERS GAME

Don't ask your wife's doctor to become "Nick the Greek" in the cancer battle. This isn't Las Vegas or Atlantic City. Often doctors are reluctant to give a figure because they could be wrong and because it could be detrimental to the patient's recovery. Why scare someone so badly that she gives up before she begins to fight?

Doctors are not crystal-ball readers. They can make educated guesses based on past cases, but that's all they are—educated guesses. If you become obsessed with the odds, you may not be able to help your wife in her recovery.

There seems to be a compulsion to ask questions that start the statistics flying. Just remember that there are variables and that there is always someone who beats the odds. Why can't it be your wife?

Naturally you're going to ask, "What are her chances?"

Suppose the reply is "Seventy percent." Now you've got the number, but what does it mean?

Most numbers are based on five-year survival rates. Don't panic. Just about everything is based on a five-year survival rate simply because once a woman has made it that long, the odds increase dramatically in her favor. Doctors will generally chart your wife's progress in one-, three-, five-, and seven-year increments with each passing year improving the odds in her favor. These are national averages and, depending on the type of cancer, your wife's recovery could be charted in shorter or longer periods.

Although talk of one, three, five, and seven years appears to be limiting, the doctors do not intend to put a limit on your wife's life. What they are telling you is that there will be time checks in her recovery process and that patients who make it to the fifth year following treatment appear to be on their way to complete recovery. If all goes well, the third year generally is the crucial year. After that they look to five years, when they will say the odds have definitely changed in your favor. They may never use the word "cured," but survival to seven and then ten years makes the odds of recurrence even more remote.

Most numbers are also based on the percentage of patients who suffer a recurrence of the disease. If your wife is given a seventy percent chance of survival, it does not automatically mean that your wife has a seventy percent chance of living five years, but that she has a seventy percent chance of cancer *not recurring* in five years. Should it recur, she will fight it again. She may live six months or a few years or decades and then be killed in a car wreck—you never know. Everything is a gamble. It's just that now you're more cognizant of the statistics, and the danger.

Bob: *We have never had what we considered to be good numbers. From the day of first diagnosis, we could tell that Martha was at high risk. The doctors wouldn't come right out and say it, but it was obvious they considered her to have a limited future. Upon reflection, I'm very pleased they did not give her an estimated life expectancy because it could have become a self-fulfilling prophecy, dousing the flickering will to live. Martha later told me that such an estimate probably would have killed her determination to fight.*

From the first day Martha's oncologist refused to be pinned down.

"What are my chances?" Martha asked him the day of the biopsy.

"Well, there's good news and bad news," he said. "The good news is that this type of cancer responds well to treatment. The bad is that it has a history of returning."

"But what are my odds?" Martha inquired again.

The doctor paused, pursed his lips, and cocked his head as if listening. It's a habit he has when considering weighty questions. It was obvious that he didn't want to reply, but Martha pressed on, forcing an answer.

"I'd say less than fifty percent," he said quietly.

"How much less?" she probed.

"That's the best I can tell you," he said.

Those horrifying odds actually looked good to us later. After three rounds of chemotherapy, we sought other opinions from a battery of doctors from the University of Texas Health Science Center. We just wanted to check and see how things were going. At that point we were also trying to decide if Martha should have the first mastectomy. Her oncologist was more than glad for us to get outside opinions.

After reviewing Martha's case, one of the doctors gave her a twenty percent chance and another a forty percent chance of the cancer not recurring. But at least she was told by one doctor that he expected her to be in the top percentile of the forty percent who made it to remission. He added that as an afterthought, basing that bit of hope on her response to treatment.

We nearly worried ourselves crazy over the statistics until Martha's oncologist gave us some very good advice.

"If it happens to you, it's a hundred percent," he told us one day when we badgered him about the odds.

It took awhile, but it finally soaked in. The doctor's point was that if a biopsy revealed cancer, then your personal chances of having cancer are a hundred percent. It doesn't matter what your statistical chances of contracting the disease *are—you've got it and accepting that fact is both difficult and key to your recovery.*

If after treatment the doctors find no evidence of cancer, you're a hundred percent free of cancer. Sure, it could come back, but odds or survival rates will not change the fact that cancer is not currently detected. From that day on you are a hundred percent cancer-free until proven otherwise.

There is another level of meaning that I find more subtle and difficult to explain. This level deals with personal perception. I think the oncologist was trying to point out that any physical or emotional incident—tragic or happy—is viewed as a hundred percent by the person experiencing it.

No matter what was going to happen in the future—good health or recurrence of the disease—it was going to be a hundred percent. So, one hundred percent became our motto.

There are many types of statistics. You almost have to be a certified public accountant to understand exactly what the numbers mean. Then when you assume they're figured out, some X-factor throws you back into a state of confusion.

It is very important to have a proper perspective in this area so as not to allow mere numbers to shake your hope. You should allow them to help when they can and regard them with some skepticism when they hurt.

In the first place, no one knows "for sure." Every medical professional will agree that there are exceptions. We know that the medical statistics in use today are the best available, but it is the word "available" that we must keep in mind.

Our society has a fairly accurate method of recording deaths, and the cause of death. Medical authorities must make an official death pronouncement and, in many cases, attending doctors sign a certificate affirming the cause of death. In cases where there is no attending doctor, an official of the medical examiner's office or the coroner's office will investigate. In suspicious cases, the medical examiner might even order an autopsy to determine the cause of death. This country has a detailed bookkeeping system to deal with the dead, and the cause of death, thereby availing researchers of a good statistical base.

The problem is that we are not nearly as good at recording life! Many women who survive cancer go on about their lives, disappearing from statistical records until their death of something other than cancer. They may eventually be killed in an accident or succumb to old age. Too often, these people—whose lives offer hope—are not part of a statistical evaluation. Statisticians do not know how long these women live or how long they remain free of cancer. Their cases could change national statistics.

Women need to know that there are thousands who defeat cancer who do not take part in surveys and who live long lives.

When it comes to statistics, we think it is wiser to ask the doctor, "Can my wife live with this?" than "Can my wife die of this?" The answer to both questions is probably "yes," but we say let the Man Upstairs set the odds. You just do your best to keep going day by day, and don't let the numbers dampen your faith in the future.

WHAT ABOUT THE POSSIBILITY OF DEATH?

While it is unpleasant, you do have to deal with the possibility of death—and the sooner, the better. Death is man and woman's ultimate challenge and you need to decide how you are going to face it. Is this going to be a time of great depression and fear, or is it going to be a time of growth and self-evaluation, for both you and your spouse? You have to attempt to work your way through this problem before you can arrive at satisfactory conclusions and the realization that there is always hope. Perhaps hope can come only after despair. A minister once told us that "No one is ever free in life until he or she has accepted their own mortality."

It may be a different type of hope than any you've ever

experienced. It may be the hope of togetherness in another world. It may be the hope of a full, wonderful life as you face the uncertainty of day-to-day living. It certainly is the hope of life together into old age, which is, after all, the first hope of a young married couple. But the hard fact remains—you have to work within the bounds of reality; so make the most of it.

If you believe in God, then turn to Him. This was our greatest refuge. If you have no belief in God, then seek out a set of humanistic principles that provide hope.

True, death is the natural order of things. But now that it could affect your wife, put yourself in her place and consider your own death, as she must now consider the possibility of hers. Decide how you might react to the news and you may view your wife in a new light. You may discover new depths of courage, determination, humor, grace, and love.

Bob: Martha had come face to face with death before, but this time the challenge seemed different. For one thing, she did not feel physically ill. That's one of the most insidious aspects of cancer. She was feeling great, her health appeared to be better than ever, and she was full of energy.

Every other serious illness in her life had been accompanied by pain, fever, chills, and general malaise. These were always followed by surgery and the struggle to survive.

This time, her reaction was a deep, absorbing depression, an understandable state considering the bad news, the impending biopsy, and the swift, debilitating dose of chemotherapy that she knew was to come.

Sensing the depth of her despair, the surgeon asked one of his longtime friends to be the anesthesiologist during the biopsy. It was a wise move. This strong-willed and compassionate woman visited Martha the night before and gave her her complete attention.

"The surgeon told me that he had a patient who needed tender loving care," she said.

She took a complete background, probed Martha's problems with nausea, and patiently explained what she would do to try to make things more bearable for her. You see, Martha has a delicate system best described as a weak stomach. Almost anything makes her ill, a problem that would really surface during chemotherapy.

"Do you want to know the biopsy results as soon as you wake up?" she asked.

"Yes," Martha replied.

The next day, instead of telling my wife she had cancer, the anesthesiologist gently said:

"Martha, you're going to have to have chemotherapy."

"I wish I had died on the operating table," Martha answered.

A realist, Martha knew what she faced. At that moment, death seemed preferable to going through chemotherapy and its devastating side effects.

The day after the biopsy, the anesthesiologist came in.

"Martha, do you remember what you told me?" she questioned, wondering if her death wish was genuine or brought on by the anesthesia.

"I remember," Martha said.

"Do you still mean it?"

"I don't know, but I sure am scared. They're going to give me the chemo in a few hours," Martha replied. "I'd almost rather do anything than be that sick."

"You'll be okay," she said, patting Martha's arm. "There are drugs to help ease the nausea."

That day, I made up my mind to let Martha talk to me about the possibility that she might die. As a concerned husband I had forced her to talk about my death by taking out life insurance and making plans to protect her. Now, it was my turn to face reality.

Talking about death has been my most difficult task. I love my wife and the thought of losing her is beyond comprehension. The only thing that has made several discussions on this topic bearable is the fact that cancer patients need to release tension and depression by talking about their feelings and fears. For this reason I decided to listen to anything Martha

*had to say, even to the point of discussing funeral arrange-
ments and our children's inheritance.*

*She was the one who broached the topic, mostly because
she's the family's financial expert, and was concerned because
I live in a financial haze. Martha carefully prepared lists:
banking affairs, insurance papers, property, bills to be paid,
etc. Ever practical, she wanted me to be prepared. She even
went on a spending spree and purchased land near Del Rio and
a condominium because "I want to be sure you're taken care
of." Due to her illness, I took over our financial affairs. "Temporarily," I told her. "If you want these things done, then you
have to get well."*

*We often shared our spiritual beliefs, discussing life after
death and drawing upon the comforting Biblical teachings that
should either of us die, we would be together again.*

*It was during this time that we had to face the deaths of
two older uncles, a dear friend, and a cousin who died of
cancer. Each incident provided a venue of discussion, especially since I spoke at the funerals of one uncle and the cousin.*

*These are difficult topics to discuss, but you'll do your
wife a favor by listening and talking. Sometimes she just needs
a sounding board to work out her fears as she clarifies her
thoughts. And, of course, there's nothing that prevents you
from pointing out how much you care for her and want her to
fight to recover.*

Every woman, and every couple, has a different way of
dealing with the possibility of death. One young woman told
a self-help group that her immediate reaction was anger—
anger that she had too much life left to live and nothing was
going to cheat her out of it.

Women have told us that they were spurred on to live
because of unfinished business: a child in high school or an
unborn grandchild. Others take a "why worry?" attitude or *que
sera sera*. But every woman with breast cancer must, at some
time, face the possibility of her own death.

This is especially difficult for women who are happily

married. A psychiatrist explained that for a happily married couple death is akin to a forced divorce or separation. After all, should she die, the wife will give up all she holds dear. And the husband, too, will lose what is most precious to him. The twist on this unique thought is that common wisdom seems to make the survivor the loser when in reality they *both* lose.

You may not know how to initiate a discussion of death. We didn't at first so we tried to let the moment dictate the direction, while remaining open to the topic. Honesty seems to be the best approach—by both husband and wife—and will get the best results.

But, should you be hesitant to tackle the issue directly, we suggest you start by discussing religion, which can always allow either of you to broach the subject of death. Be sensitive to current events. A casual remark about someone in the news—such as a right-to-die case—can be channeled into a helpful dialogue that allows either of you to reveal your thoughts on such issues as death with dignity, life-support systems, etc., without directly discussing the topic in a personal way. Sometimes a trip to a support group puts you in touch with people actually going through what you've only talked about. And, of course, there are always psychologists and psychiatrists, as well as the clergy, who offer counseling and comfort.

Ann and Andy stayed away from a straightforward discussion of death, instead they took an oblique path to the topic. It was *their* way of handling the situation.

Andy: The closest Ann and I ever came to dealing with death was one Easter Sunday when she gave us all a homemade, two-foot-by-four-foot Easter card that carried, in part, this message.

"This card is for all those with love and peace in their hearts and who believe in Him."

She signed it "Peep," one of my many nicknames for her. (As a child, she had played Little Bo Peep in the Walt Disney film classic *Babes in Toyland*.)

In my mind I had the feeling that Ann was trying to tell us

all something about how she wanted us to act with each other. I sensed that she wanted to teach us something about life before she left.

Much later, I asked her about this, after she knew she would pull through, and she denied it. She said the lesson part was right on, but not the part about "before she left."

Ann always had a great attitude about life before, during, and after cancer. We all learned from her on this point. Her attitude toward survival—both in public and private—was always upbeat.

She helped us all to think positive. Your support for your wife will grow stronger if you think positive. I learned true humility from Ann. She didn't ask "Why me?" Instead it was "Why not me?" because, she told me, "I wondered what kind of person would I be if I wished it on someone else."

Ann's favorite prayer by Saint Francis De Sales ends "Be at peace then and put aside all anxious thoughts and imaginings."

"In other words, 'Let go and let God,' " she told me.

She chalked it all up to the human condition, something that just happened, and she would make the best of her life.

Ann later confessed that she did begin to experience fear when she saw this strange look in our eyes, which she interpreted as "Oh, is this the way they look before they die of cancer."

It shook her confidence. She began to think, "Hey, maybe this thing will kill me."

The reason for her not thinking this sooner is that she has a close relative who had breast cancer more than thirty years ago. She is alive and well today. Ann thought that life always went on after breast cancer—just that you went on without a breast or two.

But when she saw that "strange look" in our eyes, she got scared. And she doubled up on her prayers.

Sometimes I believe we all have too much regard for this thing called breast cancer. It gets too much respect and should be put in its place.

Maintaining a positive attitude will be one of your more difficult tasks. You cannot let fear paralyze your functions. You'll be surprised at how much hope you can find by constantly looking for the positive in everything. If you don't live with the positive, your wife may read something into your actions that you didn't intend.

Never resign yourself to your wife's possible death. You have to be extremely careful and vigilant about this. If you resign yourself, she will sense it. She will pick up the vibrations, just as Ann began to read death in Andy's eyes. At this time, your wife will be extremely sensitive to your moods, even as you are sensitive to hers. No matter how much she knows about her situation, she may believe there is something she doesn't know: some deep, dark secret hidden from her. One man told us that sometimes the reverse happened, and he found himself wondering if his wife had told him everything the doctor had said to her. He was fearful she was trying to spare his feelings. You must keep yourself on as even a keel as possible. We know this might be a bit of a burden, but, again, consider her position.

And, finally, we learned that there are often almost unbelievable ironies in life.

Bob: *In the middle of our battle we had a special moment of grief that seemed to polarize our thoughts about death.*

Many nights the telephone would ring and a booming voice would drawl, "Whattaya doing? Why aren't you here in Del Rio playing Skipbo?" It was Bill Burk, and his wife Arlene, friends for nearly two decades; a couple as close to us as brother and sister and looked upon as a favored aunt and uncle by our children. Through personal visits, telephone calls and cards, they helped sustain us during this troublesome time.

Bill, a retired U.S. Border Patrol officer, was a man's man, equally at home in the wilderness as in his own living room. Therefore, it was a jolt one Saturday morning when we learned that Bill had drowned while on a fishing trip on the Rio Grande that also cost another life and nearly claimed two others. The men had been caught in turbulence that overturned the boat and stripped them of their lifejackets.

It was inconceivable that Bill was dead. Everyone who knew him considered him a most careful, knowledgeable man. Martha and I went to Arlene and spent several days with her, numbed by the tragedy, trying to offer her support and comfort.

On the day of the funeral, as Martha and I stood at the gravesite, she turned to me.

"I figured that if any one of the four of us was buried, it would be me," she whispered, tears coursing down her cheeks.

I understood what she meant. Of the four of us, Bill was always in better health, always the most active, and the three of us expected Bill to be going strong long after we were gone.

The point is, there are no guarantees. None of us knows what life holds in store.

As husbands we don't want our wives living under a death sentence, thinking they are about to die at any moment. Thanks to modern science, many will not die. Help her to face the *possibility* of death and keep in mind that doctors, often for legal reasons, tend to give you the worst-case scenario.

Once you have helped her learn to live with the *possibility* of death, then put that thought behind you and look forward to a wonderful future together.

Now, let's create a Life Plan.

4

Creating a
Life Plan

We encourage you to set your goal on life by taking decisive action. Prepare a "Life Plan" and make it a part of your daily living, of every decision you make and of every thought you have. Thinking in terms of life and the future will enable you to develop a more positive and confident attitude.

In the days following a cancer diagnosis, you and your wife will be forced to make some difficult decisions. Like most people, you probably have little knowledge of cancer. Until now, cancer has been a disease that happened to other people and other families, not you or your family. So at this point, you're probably better equipped to coach the Dallas Cowboys than to make some of the decisions coming your way.

Before you do anything, though, try to decide if you're happy with your doctor. How do you do that? You use your own instincts and a bit of sleuthing. Examine your emotional reaction. Is he (or she) treating you and your wife with respect? Does he answer all your questions clearly and straightfor-wardly? Does he give you enough time to even ask your questions? Then ask yourself, "How did I end up with him?" If he is a surgeon, was he recommended by your general practitioner? If an oncologist, was he recommended by your surgeon or general practitioner? Did you or your wife pick his name out of the telephone directory? Is he the right person for the job? Pick up the telephone and call the nearest medical association and ask for the background on the doctor treating your wife. The association will be glad to assist you. The association will not make recommendations, but will provide you with the doctor's educational and professional background. Be sure and ask "Is he board certified?" That means he has passed an examination designed by the American Medical Association to determine his qualifications to practice in a specified field, such as surgery. Do you know any other physicians? Call and ask them about the doctor treating your wife. If they suspect you can get better help, they will tactfully let you know.

Bob: *Don't be surprised if your surgeon or your oncologist keeps you at arm's length. They may never call you by your first name or project the same comforting warmth that flows from your family doctor, whom you've probably known for years.*

If familiarity is missing, I want to defend the doctors and give you a bit of warning. You are dealing with men or women who live under unbelievable stress. Every day they have to walk into a room and tell scared, highly excitable people that a loved one has a deadly disease. They have to watch the tears, answer the questions, and try to offer a bit of calm in a superemotional situation. On occasion they have to bear the brunt of the grief because sometimes they cannot pat you on the back and tell you that everything is going to be all right, like your family doctor can in most circumstances.

I want to be careful here. I'm not saying these highly trained doctors are uncaring; often it is the opposite, it is their deep caring that causes them to erect a barrier to protect themselves from too much emotional stress. True, there are some doctors who are cold, who tend to live in the world of mechanical medicine, and who view the patient with about the same compassion as a mechanic set to repair an automobile. But I believe these healers are in the minority.

The truth is, I did want the reassuring warmth of a personal relationship with our doctors, but more than anything I wanted them to be successful in helping my wife regain her health. If they were the best people for the job, I didn't even have to like them.

Perhaps as time goes by, and you adjust to the situation, and as your wife's condition improves, or for a number of other factors or a combination of all, you will see a change in this relationship.

Once you're happy with your doctor, take the next four basic steps preparing a Life Plan; then spend a little time reflecting.

STEP #1: GET A SECOND OPINION

And a third and a fourth and a fifth, until you are satisfied that your wife has cancer and needs immediate attention.

The doctor who diagnosed the disease will be glad to give you the names of other doctors for a second opinion. But you may want to seek out someone on your own. Like anyone else, doctors form friendships and people who think alike tend to become friends.

If you elect to try to find someone on your own, then the first place to turn is, again, the local branch of the American Medical Association. Local telephone information can provide you with the phone number of the nearest group. Keep that number handy because you may need it several times during the coming months. Get the names of several doctors and their credentials. You may want more than one second opinion.

Many full-service hospitals have added women's breast/health wings and these can be a source for a second opinion. Another source would be friends. Odds are you know someone who has gone through this ordeal; their doctor might be outstanding.

Within a couple of hours, Martha and Bob searched the

Yellow Pages, talked to a number of doctors, and quickly arranged a session with a gynecologist who treats one of Martha's bowling buddies.

"Most people get a second opinion because they don't like what they heard the first time," one doctor observed. "If the second opinion concurs with the first, then there wasn't any need of the second; but what if the second opinion differs and you find someone who tells you what you want to hear? Then you get a third opinion or a tie-breaker. That's the problem I always run into. How do you know when to stop?"

If a doctor says it's cancer, then do not be afraid to ask him or her pertinent questions, such as:

- How can you be a hundred percent sure whether it is or is not cancer?
- How big is the lump?
- Do you think she needs a biopsy?
- If she must be hospitalized and receive general anesthesia for the biopsy, will you delay treatment until she has a chance to get a second opinion on the diagnosis and proposed treatments (the two-step biopsy)?
- Why do you think it may be cancer instead of fibrocystic breast disease?
- Will my wife's health be endangered by waiting?
- What tests have you done?
- What do the results mean?
- What other tests are there and what would they tell us?
- Is it likely to spread?
- If she waits and it turns out to be cancer, will it spread to other areas?
- If she has cancer, what form of treatment would you recommend?
- Will you recommend a specialist? (If the diagnosis starts with your family doctor, he or she may recommend spe-

cialists and help you coordinate treatment. It's helpful to have a central information specialist—the family doctor—who helps guide you. Sometimes he acts as a liaison between you and the various specialists. He can interpret and explain test results. It's a good system that will help you get the ball rolling with a minimum of delay. Bob and Andy struck out on their own, and at times wished for the security of this system.)

• How about a second opinion?

You may not like the answers, but you must ask the questions. Sometimes not knowing is really worse than knowing.

Then there is the one question that doctors say they nearly always are asked, "Is it contagious?" Every doctor we've talked to assures us it is not.

If a doctor suggests a delay in treatment, find out why. Back him or her up against the wall with aggressive questions.

Sometimes a doctor will want to perform a biopsy in which a segment of the offending tissue is tested. It is the only way to be a hundred percent certain if a tumor is cancerous or benign. Get the biopsy fast and forget about the little scar and any inconvenience.

Depending on your situation, the doctor will either put your wife to sleep or excise a piece of the tumor under local anesthetic on an outpatient basis. Sometimes if the tumor is deep, a woman may go into a biopsy not knowing if she will lose her breast or not because she already has authorized the surgeon to remove the breast should cancer be discovered. Of course, she has the option of asking the surgeon to awaken her, explain the situation and test results, and reschedule another hospital visit. This is what Ann chose to do. She did not want to wake up and find her breast(s) gone.

The conditions under which your wife has a biopsy are her choice—*just be sure to get it done if necessary.*

You and your wife should use your own reasoning powers. A friend of ours did and saved her own life with the right questions. Reassured that the lump in her breast was "probably" fibrocystic and only needed monitoring, she was driving home from the doctor's office when she stopped her car on the freeway. The doctor had told her he could not be a hundred percent sure the tumor was harmless without a biopsy. Remembering Martha's and Ann's experiences, she drove back to the doctor's office and demanded to be a hundred percent sure. Biopsy proved the cyst to be not only cancerous, but also the type known as "mirror cancer." Statistics indicated that it probably would grow in the other breast; it could be weeks, months, or even years. She had a simple mastectomy to remove the contained cancer and then six weeks later had the other breast removed as a precautionary measure.

No one knows your wife and her circumstances as well as you do. So don't let a doctor's reassuring attitude keep you from following through with either a biopsy or a second opinion. Both our wives monitored the disease for a period of time and in Martha's case, it backfired. Bob and Martha lost precious time in getting the proper diagnosis and in bringing the cancer under control.

The second-opinion doctors will need to see X rays and test results. Either arrange for these to be sent to them or ask if you can carry them with you if time is critical. Do not lose these important test results and X-ray negative plates and be sure that you return them. These may become important in the future as doctors chart the progress of the illness.

Bob: I learned that lesson the hard way. The X-ray lab was willing to let me take the plates with me because Martha needed a second opinion right away. After the storm abated, I put the X-ray plates in the back of our closet and more or less forgot about them. More than a year later, Martha and I went through some rough hours because something had been discovered in her right breast and the doctors wanted to compare the current X rays with those taken earlier.

After several hours of their searching for the earlier X rays, I remembered having them and dashed home to get them.

The radiologist was now fully informed and the situation didn't look so bad as was first thought.

The doctor will ask for a number of tests. Some will be routine and others will be required because of your wife's particular case. After a physical examination the doctor will call for either standard X rays or a mammogram should he suspect a problem. The result of these tests will determine the need to monitor the lump or perform a biopsy.

A standard X ray provides a one-dimensional look at the chest area, highlighting bone and dense masses within the body, and the patient stands or lies in front of the machine. A mammogram is a more detailed look at soft tissues and is an important tool in finding cancerous tumors before they can be felt by the physician. A woman's breasts are gently compressed—pain is rare—to allow a full range of diagnostic plates. Like a standard X ray, it produces a black-and-white film plate. A xeromammography is a variation of the mammogram that produces a blue-and-white X ray on special picture. And in some instances, a doctor will call for a sonogram (sometimes called an ultrasound) in which the breasts are submerged in water (the patient leans over a container) and sound waves—similar to the sonar used by the Navy to track ships—pass through the breasts, giving diagnosticians an even more defined picture of the interior of the breast. A biopsy allows a doctor not only to check the tissue for the presence of cancer, but also to instigate a series of tests should cancer be revealed. He may ask the lab to determine if estrogen receptors are present in the affected area. The presence of such receptors could make your wife a candidate for hormonal treatment, which, in some instances, does not have the same dramatic side effects as chemotherapy. Tissue tests may also reveal the original site of the cancer.

Other tests include a chest X ray, blood count, and blood tests to check organ (liver, spleen, kidney, etc.) function. More often than not, the doctor will wait until after a positive biopsy to ask for a liver, bone, and spleen scan to determine if the cancer has spread to these areas.

Many women are paralyzed by fear and are afraid of what they'll learn from tests. So why don't you help your wife out and take the lead at this trying time?

Andy: The doctor's words echoed in my mind:

"I respect your right to get other opinions if you desire them. But I must advise you: Do not wait too long. Get the other opinions fast. . . ."

He told us that the cancer in the right breast was doubling in size at an alarming rate. The "pimple" on the left breast had been the first sign, but now the right breast was of more concern. The doctor had suggested that Ann have a mastectomy of the right breast. He also said she might be a candidate for a lumpectomy (the removal of the tumor only) on the left.

I began to form a plan. I wanted Ann to get a second opinion from scratch. My heart was fearful (and hopeful, at the same time) that he might have gotten the wrong information— like somebody else's X rays or tests results.

But to get a "pure" second opinion from scratch would mean that Ann would have to go through all the tests again.

We went for another opinion and registered under "Murcia," our married name. Ann hid her trademark blond hair and used very little makeup. My sister, Joanie, came with us.

It wasn't until the paperwork had been completed and the doctor was halfway through his checklist that he recognized Ann. He wanted to know what was going on and why she wasn't registered under her name. She explained that Murcia was her married name. He got excited that he had a celebrity in his office. At this, Ann had the nurse call me in.

I explained to the doctor that we wanted a clean second opinion, new X rays and all. He tried to talk us out of the second set of X rays, but with Ann's permission I was insistent. I explained that we wanted to make sure that those were in fact Ann's X rays being read. (My police-trained and suspicious mind was at work.)

After he put Ann through a new series of tests, the doctor again explained that he could have studied the X rays taken of Ann by the other radiologist and saved time, money, and extra radiation. Maybe I was being too careful, but if you can't sleep at night from worrying, get that second round of tests; however, I would not recommend that you go as far as I did because of the extra expense in time and money and the low-dosage radiation. The only real justification for taking new X rays and tests is if the X ray is not so clear as it could be or if you have reasonable grounds to believe that the X rays being read are not your wife's.

When we had gotten the extra assurance that we needed, it was time for the news.

The doctor recommended that both of Ann's breasts be removed, but he felt that she would survive.

I looked at Ann.

"Come on," she said, rising swiftly. Her body seemed supercharged with energy. "Let's get out of here while the rest of me is still intact." It might have been a "Cassie" one-liner, but I knew what was going on in that sweet head.

She marched straight out of the building and began walking swiftly down the street as I followed, trying to talk to her. Ann spotted one of those gaudy, youth-oriented bluejean stores featuring rock 'n' roll music and flashing strobe lights. To my amazement, Ann went in and walked right up to a rack of some of the most outlandish clothes I've ever seen and began to go through them, yanking each item to one side after a quick glance.

"Ann, I don't think you want to buy any of these . . ." I started.

"I'm doing just fine," she snapped, not looking up, appearing to be totally absorbed in clothing she normally wouldn't give a second look.

A young saleswoman came up. She had yellowish hair atop reddish-green makeup and her appearance was just as outlandish as the place.

"How ya doin'? Need any help?" she asked.

"I'm doing just fine," Ann told her in the same courteous but no-nonsense voice she had used with me.

Sensing that this customer wasn't in a normal frame of mind, the clerk retreated.

I walked up and gently took her arm, stopping her frantic search.

"Ann."

"I'm dealing with it in my own way," she said, looking up, her eyes moist. "I'm trying to find a little bit of relief."

Then, one of the personal demons that would plague her throughout the ordeal escaped:

"How am I going to tell Mama and Papa?" she whispered.

My heart went out to her. She had just received terrible news and her concern was her parents, not herself. We were to pick them up in a couple of hours for dinner.

On the drive home, we stopped and took a long walk on the beach, holding hands, each absorbed in our own thoughts.

"We won't tell my parents tonight. We'll wait until after the weekend and . . ." she paused. "Andy, *I* want to tell them. I don't want anyone else to."

I understood. They are elderly and she wanted to soften the blow as much as possible.

That night, Ann put on the performance of her life. Her parents never suspected a thing and when the four of us drank a toast to life, Ann and I exchanged a meaningful look.

It was a long weekend, waiting to talk to the original doctors, making arrangements for the surgery, and taking that first bold step to recovery and life. We had our second opinion. We knew what to do. It was time to act.

Do not delay in getting a second opinion and initiating treatment. Would you live in a home with a time bomb on the coffee table? Of course not! Breast cancer is a ticking bomb and just as deadly; maybe even more so because it attacks silently. A delay in treatment could mean death or rapid spread of the disease.

You will be surprised at how most surgeons and oncologists (doctors who specialize in cancer treatment) not only recommend, but also insist on a second opinion. They welcome help. But always pay attention to the timetable they set.

And if by chance you find yourself with a doctor who resists second opinions or discourages them, then drop him or her like a hot potato. The only thing such a physician might suffer is a bruised ego, while you might lose your wife.

STEP #2: PARTICIPATE, PARTICIPATE, PARTICIPATE

Andy: If I have learned one thing from all this, it is that us guys had better always take a keen interest in our wife's health.

In my case, prior to my going with Ann to the doctor's office when things started looking bad, I had been letting my sister, Joanie, take Ann to her regular doctor's appointments. It was routine.

So, when I started seeing my sister and wife whispering a lot at home, I became suspicious. It took a few questions before they admitted to me that they were "watching" something and just did not want to worry me. That's when I got involved. I wish I had gotten involved sooner, like three months sooner.

My mistake was not involving myself in the most routine matters; after all, your wife is the woman you love and your partner in life.

And I have a message to wives, also. Don't shut out your husband in these matters, especially now. We know you don't want to worry him unnecessarily, but it's better for him to be in on it from the start.

Like Bob, I will always wonder if my not being involved early caused the cancer to stay when it could have been removed three months earlier.

Don't hesitate. Don't wait, especially if something shows up later in the other breast. By then you know the drill: swift, sure action.

Participation is the linchpin in the Life Plan. We put participation second only because it is of primary importance to secure immediate treatment. You may not have the knowledge, the technical expertise, or the ability to medically assist your wife, but you do have something that is extremely important to her emotional well-being: your love, your presence, and your participation.

Doctors can tell you numerous horror stories about distraught and frightened women trying to make life and death decisions while their husbands sat, mum, listening but not contributing anything to the decision-making process.

We will never be accused of being shy, so it seemed only natural for us to jump in. But even if it doesn't seem natural for you, remember that your wife needs your support now more than ever, especially if she is being forced to take what might be an unpleasant stance (switching doctors, getting second opinions) that could compound her stress.

Some wives have told us that their husbands refused to talk to them about their cancer, almost as if they believed that by ignoring it, the problem would go away. Some husbands don't want to listen, they don't want to consider unpleasant possibilities. It's true that some women withdraw and tend to keep their own counsel. But most women in this situation have a need to talk, to think outloud. So listen. Try to understand, to get into her mind as you participate in her healing. Help her to make decisions while respecting her right to make the ultimate decision.

Your wife is in a weakened condition now. Before treatment she faces a desperate mental struggle. Afterward it is compounded by the physical battle. So try to help bolster her spirits with a quiet dinner at a favorite restaurant, or a bouquet of flowers "Just because I love you," or a few hours "to do anything you want," or a leisurely back rub or a restoring ride in the countryside. Andy and Ann would go to the beach and feed the seagulls, soaking up the sunshine and natural beauty, often using this change of scene as an opportunity to discuss hard medical decisions.

At this particular time, you may be the only one capable of gathering and assessing the facts. Be sure you understand as much as possible—even if it means arranging private talks with the doctor that could tear your guts out. Then, try to make sure your wife understands everything. Neither of you needs any surprises.

Sharpen your memory, take notes. You'll be amazed at how often you misunderstand, so don't hesitate to jot things down. Ask plenty of questions and don't be afraid to tell the doctor when you don't understand something. Keep listening and talking until you do. Many times your wife will rely on your memory when fear and anxiety cloud her own.

Andy: If I had it to do over, I'd buy a notebook at the start and use it as a diary to enter every doctor's visit and every procedure suggested or performed, plus the date, time, and anything else I might need to check later. What a help that would have been.

I started keeping notes and dates after a while and now I keep a record of everything. It works for me because I don't like to have the doctor pulling my coat when another exam is due. It's a way of taking control of one's own health.

Several husbands have since told me that they take a small tape recorder into sessions with their doctors.

Most couples establish areas of expertise during their years of marriage; sometimes one spouse will dominate the relationship. Household chores, day-to-day operations, child rearing, financial records, home care tend to come under the control of the spouse who is particularly suited to that task or is willing to accept that particular responsibility. Falling loosely under this category is the job of information gathering. It doesn't matter who performed that function in the past—now it is *your* job. If your wife wishes to continue as the information gatherer, that's even better because two heads are better than one; but you now need to take a more active role.

STEP #3: BECOME INFORMED
ABOUT THE DISEASE

Knowledge is power. Read and talk. Learn everything you can. You might not like some of what you learn, but you need knowledge to combat cancer. You may find that the first gleaning of knowledge will scare you more than enlighten you, but as you become more informed about the disease, the treatments, the medical terms, and the help available, you will discover that it is certainly not always a hopeless battle. And with that discovery comes a measure of confidence.

Bob: I'd like to say a word about the "worst-case scenario." Until I finally grasped its real meaning—and purpose— I spent many hours in fear.

Several days before Martha was scheduled for her first mastectomy, her surgeon seemed to change a bit from his usual warm, comforting, and engaging style. Suddenly, he was telling us about all the terrible things, including death, that could happen to her. After a while, he turned to his nurse and asked:

"Have I said enough to fulfill the law?"

She nodded and the doctor walked out, leaving a badly shaken couple. Was Martha going to live or die? What about all these bad things?

Later, a doctor from the University of Texas Health Science Center would do the same thing, only this time he would use the words "worst-case scenario." I finally came to understand that, for legal reasons, doctors have to tell you the worst that could happen. I began to listen for that phrase and to realize that the doctors did not mean these things would necessarily happen to Martha but that they were the worst possible eventualities. And because the "worst-case scenario" generally deals with suffering and death, it tends to dominate your thoughts, rather than the encouragement they may have just offered.

We know that getting a crucial second opinion first and then starting to educate yourself on the subject seems to be putting the cart before the horse. But, in truth, most people don't have the luxury of studying cancer before making difficult decisions.

And until your knowledge increases, you will find yourself in a dilemma: You need to make a crucial decision and you realize the knowledge you have is woefully inadequate. At this point, your best source of knowledge is the doctor. Draw on his or her experience. Also, talk to everyone: nurses, therapists, and friends or acquaintances who have fought the battle. Telephone the American Cancer Society or the cancer information group nearest you for information on specific questions. (Also see the "Selected Reading" and "Resources" sections, beginning on page 209 of this book.)

Another important source of knowledge can be the many self-help and support groups for women with breast cancer that can be found at hospitals and treatment centers. Some groups are open to family participation, encouraging the husband, children, and relatives of women with breast cancer to attend weekly meetings at which common problems are discussed. Other groups are reserved for the women themselves or for women and their spouses.

If your wife is hesitant, it would be a good idea for you to attend a meeting of a self-help group, alone. You can judge if such sessions will help her. You will have to be sensitive to her mental condition should you urge her to attend one of these groups. Forcing her to go against her will could do more harm than good. It should be *her* choice. Should she decide not to go, you may want to attend on your own. You might find it helpful to talk to a fellow soldier in the cancer battle. And don't overlook the obvious advantage of such a support group: You meet people who are success stories—people you both need to know.

Bob: Martha and I have had little to do with organized groups. They don't fit her personality and approach to survival.

"I don't have anything in common with those women," Martha told me one day after I made her visit a mastectomy group.

"But you're soon going to lose a breast," I rejoined. "Maybe you could learn from them."

"I'm not interested right now," she said, her offhand response belying deep-rooted feelings that would eventually erupt in a fit of anger.

"I'm tired of being considered a victim," Martha told me months later. "I've had cancer. I've had a mastectomy and I've survived. I try not to live with it in my thoughts every day. I want to treat it like any other illness, put it behind me, and forget it," she fumed. "I don't want people looking at me and thinking 'that's the woman who had cancer.' They wouldn't do it if they knew you had had the flu or chicken pox."

We never went to another group meeting. It would have been grossly unfair to force her to go. She would have gone had I insisted, knowing that I was motivated by love, but it would have done more harm than good.

Each woman must deal with this in her own way.

But each man must deal with it in his way, too, and if you would feel better attending one of the many support groups, then do so.

Me? I would gladly embrace the camaraderie of such a group.

And, of course, nothing informs you better than good, hard study. Both of us have amassed a library of books on cancer, plus newspaper and magazine articles, along with numerous brochures. We also cherish our many inspirational books that have buoyed our spirits and given us hope.

We sat up many a night into the wee hours reading everything we could get our hands on. Time consuming? You bet it was; but it later proved invaluable in understanding our wives' cases. It is our intent that this knowledge be passed on through this book, and you can catch up on the sleep we missed.

You will be pleased to discover that as your knowledge increases, so will your resolve, and together they will help lessen your fears. As you and your wife gain knowledge of and familiarity with the disease, it becomes a bit easier to function, to make the difficult decisions. Even bad news is put into perspective as you gain strength—and confidence—through knowledge.

Andy: When Ann went into the hospital for her biopsy, she registered with an older woman, who had been brought in by

her son. My sister, Joanie, her husband Fred, and I hung out with him in the waiting room.

Some hours later, the son was told that the results of his mother's tests were negative. She did not have breast cancer. He jumped for joy and we congratulated him. When his mom was wheeled out, we told her how happy we were for her. She and Ann had gone through the preliminary stuff together and Ann wished her good luck and God's blessings. The woman responded with a heartfelt *l'chaim,* to life, as her son wished us *mazel tov,* good luck. The lady was very excited about having gone through this with Ann Jillian beside her. When she left she patted my hand and said: "I saw such a good heart in your wife that I feel sure God will take care of her, no matter what."

Shortly after this I spotted Ann on a gurney, being wheeled into a small room. I almost went through the glass-paneled door, but caught myself, knowing it was off limits. Ann looked so bad—her childlike face was chalk white and none of her hair was showing. I was devastated for her.

This was the first time I had seen Ann in a hospital setting. It scared me so much that I got this nauseous feeling in the pit of my stomach. An orderly who had been with her came out the door. I stopped him to ask about Ann and all he would tell me was that Ann was resting comfortably now and that the doctor would be out soon to give us the details.

For the second time, I knew it was bad news. The doctor told us that Ann definitely had cancer. I lost track of whatever else he said and stared at the floor.

I think I learned every line in that floor tile. And each line reminded me of that long, long road Ann had traveled in her young life to earn the financial security that had allowed her to take care of her elderly parents. Did this news mean that she might now be traveling a shorter road? A young life so full of love. A young life always willing to give a smile and a kind word to all she passed.

Ann's original diagnosis, the second opinion, and now the confirming biopsy left no doubt. The doctor was giving it to me right between the eyes. I was almost in walking shock, but then something special happened. I paused, suddenly realizing that I was staring at the floor, my mind wandering in an attempt to escape the reality of the moment. I refocused my thoughts, forcing the knowledge I had gleaned over the past few weeks to the fore. I knew there was hope. I knew it would be a tough battle and it was now time to start.

I looked up at the doctor, then started talking. This time it wasn't rage, but rather experience and knowledge laced with confidence that came through.

"Okay, Doc. What's the next step? What do I do to help Ann, and when will you go back in and remove her breasts?" I asked. There was no question in my mind that her breasts would be removed.

Joanie told me later that the doctor realized that I had nearly gone into walking shock. He repeated his advice that both breasts must come off. There was no chance for a lumpectomy.

"Well, we've had our second opinion and now our biopsy. It's time to get on with it," I said.

When she knew for sure that both breasts had to be removed to save her life, Ann became more determined to follow through than I had ever seen her before. Being the lover of life that she is, there was not much more to discuss after she said, "Okay, we know what we have to do, and even though I'm going to miss my breasts, living my life is more important."

"Is there anything else we can do that you know of before we do this? I just want to be sure we're not overlooking another solution," I asked.

"I wish there were, but I really feel that this is our only option," she responded, her voice faltering slightly. "I . . . I . . . I want to cry so bad."

"Go ahead," I said as I gently took her into my arms. "And I hope you don't mind if I join you."

Ann placed her head on my chest and we both cried, our tears intermingling. My grief for her was so great that it was almost impossible to concentrate, but self-control fought to the surface as I realized that Ann was trying to talk through her tears.

"I think, way back in my head, I was kind of expecting it. Don't ask me why, I just knew one day this would happen to me."

(One time Ann had inadvertently walked in on a close relative on her mother's side of the family and discovered that the woman had had a mastectomy.)

"Since then, I just kind of expected it to happen to me. I wish it were all a nightmare and that this was not really happening to us, Andy." She looked at me ruefully and, as every wife has done at one time or another, posed the fearful question.

"Are we going to be all right?"

"You bet we are, babe. Nothing could come between us, and besides," I said, drawing on my best Humphrey Bogart impersonation, "nobody quits the mob, until I say so. You're stuck with me!"

This time she didn't laugh as in the past, but I settled for a tiny smile forced through her tears. It was the best she could muster under the circumstances.

"That's my girl," I comforted. "Wait and see. Everything will be just fine and we will get through this, just like we've gotten past all the other rocks in our roadway."

It was one of our favorite metaphors. We considered obstacles to be "rocks in the roadway," and we always talked about getting out of the car and moving them out of our way so that we could go on with whatever we were doing.

Ann needed one more bit of reassurance as she began to wind down her cry.

"Ours is the love we were both searching for, isn't it?" she asked me.

"Yes" was my simple reply.

"We will fight for it and I will come out of this okay and we will be together," she said, giving a positive accent to the word "will."

"That's an order," I barked in my best ex-police sergeant voice that I sometimes use to tease Ann.

She looked up at me and finally managed to smile a real smile and we hugged, our faces sloppy with tears. There was a great deal of peace in just hugging, our arms locked around each other for what seemed like forever.

As I was holding Ann, touching her, I realized what to me is a great truth. We were nourishing ourselves through the comfort of touch, as though as long as we were holding each other, we could not be separated. Suddenly the joyous act of hugging took on this entirely new meaning, different than at any time we had ever held each other before. We were safe in each other's arms and it felt good because we needed that feeling so much.

STEP #4: REMEMBER YOUR FAMILY'S NEEDS

Sometimes you just assume that everything is understood by the family. But if *you* are confused and you're living in the middle of the tornado, think how others must feel when they receive all their information secondhand. Take time to visit with your family—especially your children—and clearly answer all of their questions. Be as honest as possible. If you don't know something, admit it; make a note of the question and find out the answer. To admit you don't know something can sometimes be reassuring to your family because you may discover they harbor the same suspicion as your wife: the fear that you are hiding information or the "true situation." On several occasions, one of Bob's children would ask, "Are you telling me everything?" Sometimes if Bob got a little down, one of the youngsters would ask, "Is there something I don't know?"

Often these family exchanges will provide you with questions that help you prepare for the next session with the doctor.

Your children may need special attention. This is an especially trying time for them no matter what their age. Unless they are extremely young, they probably were at the hospital with you the day of surgery. They probably heard the doctor explain the situation.

The very young need positive reassurance. They can help their mother pack for the hospital visit. The length of stay should be estimated with an explanation that it could be shorter or longer. Point out that when mother gets home she will be healing and not performing her normal chores. Above all, stress that a hospital is a place of healing and treatment. Also stress that mother *will* return home, no matter what the results. Should the disease advance, then handle each hospital stay within the context of the situation. Everything that will be done at the hospital should be explained at their level of understanding. Today's youngsters are extremely sophisticated, so this shouldn't be a difficult task.

Before and after treatment, remember that children take pride in being able to help. It makes them feel important and their participation helps relieve anxiety because they are helping their mother to get well again. Being included in the battle plan can help ward off a trio of unfortunate emotions that sometimes hit: fear, a feeling of worthlessness, and blaming themselves for their mother's illness.

Some families routinely hold "family councils" on decisions that affect everyone. If you've never held one, it might be a good time to give it a try. It would certainly draw everyone into the fray, each person contributing his or her thoughts to the game plan, and becoming an integral part of the support team. Such a meeting would help you establish new individual responsibilities as the family unit undergoes temporary changes because of the mother's illness. By each of you sharing the load, it may draw you closer together as a family. Finally, and more importantly, such an outpouring of love and concern and family cooperation couldn't help but give mother's spirits a boost.

Remember that your wife's family may be just as shell-shocked as you. It is up to you to take the lead in putting any personal family differences aside, should they exist. The last thing your wife needs is conflict between you and your in-laws.

Now is the time for everyone to pull together. Keep them informed of everything. It would be cruel to leave them guessing concerning her condition and treatment plan. They need to be involved in everything.

And don't forget your family—or her in-laws. As with her family, it is your responsibility to set aside family differences, should they exist. Of course they probably love her as another daughter and you know they are concerned about you and the children. So keep your family fully informed, also.

Bob: *The burden proved almost more than our daughter could bear. Martha became ill during Liländ's senior year in high school. Although we have always been a close family, when Martha's illness struck, Liländ, then seventeen, tended to withdraw into herself, almost denying that her mother was seriously ill. She seldom talked about it.*

Then one night something awoke me shortly after midnight. We were used to late-night activities, as our home has always been a haven for our children's friends. But there had been no visitors that night and when I checked the house, I discovered that Liländ was missing and the front door unlocked.

I awakened her brother and we searched the house and surrounding yards. By now Martha had awakened.

"Is there anywhere she might go?" I asked.

"To her boyfriend's house," my son Bobby offered, but I pointed out that her car was still here.

We decided to check anyway in case she had called him and he had picked her up. The motor of his car was cold, so we decided to search the neighborhood. By now it was nearing two A.M. and the three of us were even more alarmed.

Bobby and I flagged down a police officer. San Antonio has more than its share of weird incidents and it seemed possible to us that someone might have abducted her from the house. At any rate, it was out of character for Liländ to just get up and leave without telling us. We were genuinely concerned.

As Bobby and I drove back to the house—the officer fol-
lowing to make out a report—we met Lilánd riding with Cindy
Wulf, a neighbor and family friend. Lilánd had walked over to
Cindy's house, awakened her, and talked to her for several
hours because she felt the need for an adult shoulder other
than her parents'. I had not found the note Lilánd had left on
her pillow.

We were so relieved to find her safe.

Like our daughter, our son pretty much kept his own coun-
cil. It wasn't until months later that I realized what Bobby,
twenty-one, had gone through during those early days of treat-
ment.

He was in the second semester of his freshman year in
dental school at the University of Texas Health Science Cen-
ter, which happened to be across the street from the hospital
where his mom was receiving treatment. One of his required
courses was gross anatomy in which students dissect cadav-
ers.

"It seemed like every cadaver had died of cancer of some
sort," he told me rather ruefully.

Can you imagine what emotional trauma our son suffered
in silence each time he would leave the gross anatomy labora-
tory to visit his mother?

It will help ease family tension if you strive to keep everyone informed on the day of biopsy, surgery, or treatment.
Before you go to the hospital or treatment center, get a small
notebook and record everyone's telephone number, especially
long-distance numbers with area codes. In Martha's case, the
majority of her relatives were notified by long distance. A
single telephone call to her brother took care of her Dallas
relatives. Her brother passed the word on to aunts, nephews,
and nieces. A single telephone call to Bob's parents took care
of that side of the family.

Ann's parents, who live nearby, were told of her illness at
a backyard barbecue at the Murcias'.

Andy: I knew what this would do to Ann's elderly parents but she couldn't protect them from it any longer. She made the decision to tell them herself, privately.

As was her custom, Ann walked her mom and dad past the pool, toward her favorite part of the garden. They had a ritual they liked to follow. Ann would show off her flowers and her dad, Joe, would tell her of the happy times when he was a young farm boy prior to World War II. Joe would then tell Ann that she had inherited his green thumb. Her mother, Margaret, would nod in agreement.

They are a happy, close family. Joe and Margaret fled Lithuania with Ann's older brother perched on the front of a bicycle. It was rough on them when they arrived in this country. Joe was a pilot who attended the Lithuanian version of the Air Force Academy but was reduced to taking any job to support his family. He eventually became a highly skilled machinist, crafting medical equipment. The family never forgot their roots and Ann was reared speaking Lithuanian. There was always laughter and happiness in their lives, no matter what.

But not today. As I watched Ann talk to them, I saw Joe stamp his foot in anger and shock and pull out his handkerchief and begin to cry. He had a shocked look on his face and across the way I could hear a muffled, "Jesus, oh Jesus, our Jesus, help us" in his best broken English. Margaret and Ann were hugging and Joe joined them, all three hugging and crying.

In a few minutes they seemed to settle down because Ann told them it had been caught early and everything would be okay. Joe stressed that "something bad inside must come out fast." Ann spoke to them again and they calmed down more. Soon they walked back. Ann wanted to tell them alone because she was worried that they would be confused if too many people spoke to them at once.

TAKE TIME TO THINK

From time to time, find yourself a quiet spot and take a moment to reflect. If you can't find a quiet spot, then utilize the time it takes to drive to work. You need a bit of privacy for some good old-fashioned cogitation. You need to consider the emotional state of both you and your wife, the progress of the battle, and your next step in bringing her along to full health. It's during these quiet times you can write down questions (if you're not driving a car), apply your newfound knowledge to the problem at hand, and consider what little surprises, gifts, etc., you can spring on your wife to make her day a bit more pleasant.

Think about your family. What about the other women in you life? Now that your wife has breast cancer, it might be a good idea to have teenage daughters checked and taught proper breast self-examination techniques because statistics show that breast cancer can be hereditary. How about your wife's mother and sisters and aunts and female cousins? Encourage them to get a checkup.

Consider, also:

- Is the doctor treating your wife as an individual, carefully tailoring the treatment to her needs, or is the doctor using "standard" treatments?

- Are you comfortable with the doctors and their choice of treatments?

- Are the doctors knowledgeable about the latest developments in breast cancer treatment?

- Have you turned to the proper resources for help? Doctors, treatment centers, hospitals, etc., have informational pamphlets and can put you in touch with resource groups.

- Have you explored the options to your wife's satisfaction and to your satisfaction?

- And, finally, just how important are her breasts to you?

We leave you with only a few hints as to what to do with this time because we encourage you to think about what is unique to your situation.

5

Deny the Nay-Sayers

If you haven't met a "nay-sayer" yet, you will. This is the well-meaning friend who insists on giving you or your wife a blow-by-blow account of someone he or she knew who died of cancer. It's strange, but people seem compelled to tell cancer patients these horror stories. Generally they start the conversation by inquiring about your wife's health, then they try to "top" anything you or she tells them. These people may be difficult for you to take, but they are devastating for your wife. Both you and she know full-well that people can die of cancer. Your aim is positive thinking, to make that your goal.

Andy: Many people, including coworkers, tried to relate to Ann's problem with "horror stories" that were always about people who had breast cancer; people who always died; and in dying they always suffered such pain that no medicine could even ease it.

"Oh, yes," they would say.

"My friend was thirty-five years old when she got it." (The same age as Ann.)

"Her lymph nodes were clear, too." (Just as Ann's were.)

"She had one of the best, most positive mental outlooks I've ever seen." (Just as Ann does.)

"But she died, poor thing." (But not Ann.)

It was as if these people were trying to take away all of Ann's weapons in this battle; leave her defenseless; break down hope.

But Ann's faith in God and her "home team" of people who love her kept her pumped up.

Whenever I heard this, or saw it coming, I stepped in.

Nay-sayers also take the form of well-meaning friends or family who decide your wife "must" face the reality of the situation and then graphically discuss everything that has happened or could happen.

Sometimes you can switch the conversation to the "positive": good news from test results, how fortunate you are in having a thoughtful doctor, nurses, etc., or improvements in your wife's condition.

But you have to be firm with these people. It is best to change the subject if a depressing story begins; interrupt if you have to to switch to a topic of common interest. The weather is always a good, safe subject. Everyone has noticed if it's too hot or too cold or a beautiful spring day. It wouldn't hurt to prepare a mental list of several subjects that interest your wife and keep them in mind while around other people. It can be anything: a new plant in her garden, a movie she recently saw, your children's grades, a new dress, or even politics. But if that nay-sayer keeps returning to an unpleasant topic, and you have to be rude, be rude.

Andy: On occasion, I was forced to use what Ann calls my "Andy belly bounce" to rescue her from a difficult situation.

The first time I used it, Ann was being held hostage by a rude drunk who was blowing cigarette smoke in her face while mouthing some nonsense about how cancer was a "death wish" of those who did not eat right (like he did) and who were overweight (like I was). Trust me. The guy was a goofball. I tried everything. I suggested that Ann and I dance, but still he hung on, even when I said the tune was my favorite love song. You couldn't change the topic of conversation because he insisted on returning to cancer.

Finally, I had had enough. I eased up to the guy and pinned him against the wall with my big stomach while putting on one of my biggest smiles. To the world, it appeared that two buddies were face to face, planning a fishing trip. In reality, I was talking tough through my smile.

"If you don't stop telling cancer horror stories to my wife, I'm going to let this big belly of mine squash you right now. So, put on a big smile and let's talk baseball, man!"

The nay-sayer is perhaps one of the most startling revelations of this battle. In utter amazement, man after man has told us that they were forced to be rude, often asking a visitor to go home. So, if you have to ask someone to stop visiting your wife, then do so—you won't be the first husband to take that action. Sometimes this even cuts across family lines and causes strained relations, but your wife's emotional well-being should be your first concern.

What you want is good news, good times, and good health. There are thousands of success stories of people who beat cancer. Find them and surround your wife with them instead of with nay-sayers. It's the old belief in the power of positive thinking. If your wife hears only about failure, she might give up. We are dealing with unknown factors—"X-factors" if you will—that could make a difference in treatment. Laughter, lightheartedness, and contentment are what she needs, not depressing, gloom-and-doom stories.

Bob: Although we both love drama, we deliberately changed our television and movie-viewing habits for more than a year.

We seldom saw anything but comedies during Martha's illness. We didn't care how good or bad. They were Disney movies, slapstick, anything just to make us laugh or be filled with the warmth of human kindness. Modern sitcoms tend to be preachy or deal with serious subjects in a lighthearted way. We found escape in some of the classics from the past—Jack Benny, Lucille Ball, and George Burns and Gracie Allen were some of the comedians we watched in reruns—and Martha especially liked "Gilligan's Island," "Mr. Ed," and "My Three Sons." There is a gentle humor here that pokes fun at mankind's foibles without today's frenetic pacing.

The late Jackie Gleason is one of Martha's favorite comedians and I bet she knows every routine ever done by the Great One. She even taped a number of them and watched them over and over. These, by far, were her favorites.

We are still very choosy about topics.

You know your wife better than anyone in the world. Make it your responsibility to help keep her world happy. We're not talking about the same gut-busting happiness that comes from big events such as Christmas, etc., but the small, everyday joys that relieve tension.

Whenever Ann writes to women who are depressed, she always tells them to just try standing in front of a mirror and try hard to smile; or better yet, laugh. It is good therapy to laugh. We're the first to admit that while women are recovering from surgery that they have every right to cry, but laughter does the body—and the soul—so much good.

A sense of humor can be one of your more important assets in the battle against cancer. Laughter is contagious so look for it in everything you do. And savor those warm private jokes that you share as a couple.

You *can* laugh, even when going through these difficult times. Often a smile will lead to tension-releasing laughter that can neutralize a potentially painful incident.

Andy: Laughter saved the day the first time Ann went swimming after her surgery. It had been months since the operation and we had taken all of her favorite swimsuits to a special shop to have them refitted to her new figure.

On the day of her first swim, Ann came out of the house with a T-shirt over her suit. She quickly slipped into the water, but only up to her waist. I was already in the pool and I urged Ann in further, but she hesitated. I sensed her getting down in the dumps so I decided to make her laugh by flipping off my bathing suit and mooning her. But still she held back. We had often played like this, but Ann was reluctant this day.

"I'll give you my bathing suit if you'll come into the water and play," I teased.

This brought tears. I hugged and comforted Ann before I realized what was happening. In the past on occasions like this, I would sneak up and untie the top of her swimsuit while she tried to squirm away. Now Ann felt that our little game was gone forever.

Well, I soon fixed that. I went underwater and pinched her firmly on the backside, just enough to get her mad as a hornet. She started to chase me. I let her catch me and she held me under the water so long I thought I was done for. The telephone rang, saving me, and I leapt from the pool to answer it. I forgot that I didn't have my bathing suit on and that sight tickled Ann's funnybone. She started laughing.

"You look like an egg rolling down the street on a skateboard," she taunted.

She was right. I weighed about two hundred sixty pounds at the time and there was a *big* moon out. But I'll do anything to get my lady to laugh when she feels blue. Moments of "down time" are to be expected but a good laugh goes a long way in relieving tension. So keep your sense of humor, especially where your wife is concerned.

Humor often arises even in the bleakest of situations and there are many women around the country who have used a good sense of humor to get themselves over the top. Ann and Andy received an original poem in the mail from just such a lady and Ann now uses this poem in her lectures. The poignant work never fails to bring down the house with applause, a few tears and, yes, hearty laughter because it encapsulates many

of the emotions and problems we've dealt with, and does so
with a wry sense of humor.

UNTITLED
By Sylvia Riveness

They tell me that it's cancer,
    that the breast has got to go.
My anger makes me throw things
    and the tears won't stop their flow.

I question all the doctors
    and I plow through every book
'Cause I know I'll find their error
    if I study and I look.

But at last I come to realize
    that the doctors all are right
And I have to bite the bullet
    and to overcome my fright.

The telephone keeps ringing—
    It's my family and friends
who tell me of their sorrow
    and the prayers that they send.

Tomorrow's Operation Day.
    It's time to say goodbye
To a friend that's been a part of me—
    a thing that made men sigh!

I know it's kind of silly
    talking to a mound of fat
But we've shared a lot together
    and you're more to me than that.

You've been my sign of femaleness,
    my sexiness and style.

You've dictated my image
*   and held up for quite a while.*

From groping teen-age "cop-a-feels"
*   to college frat pre-meds,*
To loving, caring marriage strokes
*   and pillowed babies' heads.*

Thank you for a job well-done;
*   when needed you were there.*
I don't fault you for breaking down;
*   just for breaking up a pair!*

I can't tell Mom and Dad just yet,
*   the shock would be too much.*
I'll tell them when it's over
*   then I'll keep in constant touch.*

It's D-Day and I'm in OR
*   and suddenly start to sob*
When I see the lights and masks and know
*   it's time to start the job.*

I say goodbye and drift away
*   and next thing that I know*
I hear a voice say, "Here she comes"
*   and, "Sylvia, wiggle your toe."*

The first day is a haze of fog
*   and I'm feeling pretty bad.*
My stomach won't stop churning
*   and my head's a cotton pad.*

My bathroom habits save me
*   'Cause who else do you know*
that every minute has to walk
*   from bed to bath to go?*

The next day I'm in great shape
*   with makeup all in place.*

The IV's gone; I'm getting bored;
*   but bed's still my home base.*

The flowers and the candy
*   and the friends who come to say*
"My God, I can't believe how great
*   you look in just one day."*

My doc (I think I love him) smiles
*   "You need have no more fear.*
The lymph nodes say they're negative
*   so now you're in the clear."*

Today I'm back at home again;
*   it's just a memory.*
But I've got a flat reminder
*   of what was done to me.*

I've got a great big luncheon date
*   set up with all my friends.*
We're gonna laugh and eat and drink
*   and pat the waiters' ends.*

And then we're going shopping
*   to find a new foam breast.*
They'll tell me if it's pointy
*   and can pass the pinching test.*

We'll pick one that looks perfect
*   so that when I strut my stuff*
I'll still get looks and whistles
*   from the guys who think they're buff.*

So outside I'll be different
*   And with changes some will see*
But if you look way down inside
*   you'll see that I'm still ME!*

(reprinted with permission from the author)

6

The Physical Battle

There is a computer game in which row after row of fanciful satellites attack a home base. It is the player's challenge to dash back and forth across the bottom of the screen using a single cannon to destroy the attackers. There are various shields behind which you can hide to avoid incoming rounds. Several options make the game more difficult: it can be programmed so that the invaders zigzag instead of attacking in a straight line so you don't know exactly where the satellites will hit; and the invaders and their missiles can become invisible. The player dashes madly about, firing missiles at a blank screen, trying to avoid unseen enemy fire—all the while watching his shields disappear as the enemy artillery eats them up. The player fires as many times as he can and runs for his life. He knows he's been successful when he sees the flash caused by the destruction of an enemy satellite.

In many ways, that's what fighting breast cancer is like. Even doctors agree that cancer treatment is often an inexact science, although everything they do is based upon exacting study and research. It is a puzzle: Sometimes two women with similar problems will react differently to the same medication.

One woman may become violently ill as a result of chemotherapy while another may be only mildly nauseous. One woman's cancer may begin to disappear while the other's continues to grow. This disease is unlike anything you've ever experienced, so be patient as the doctor tries to explain various treatments. Ask questions and remember to take notes. If there is something you'd like to discuss privately, then by all means call the doctor and set up an appointment. You need to have as clear an understanding as possible. Above all, we urge you to remember that your wife is an individual and requires individual treatment.

Our wives are good examples of individual treatment. Martha had chemotherapy, radiation, and then surgery. Ann had surgery and then chemotherapy. Bear in mind that the order of specific medical treatment our wives received might not be proper for your wife but certain generalities do exist in treatment.

The modern medical community comes closer every day to discovering the "magic missile" that will attack only cancer cells, leaving the rest of a person's body unaffected. But until that time comes, cancer continues to be treated primarily by surgery, radiation, chemotherapy, or a combination of any or all of these.

DEFINING CANCER

As laymen, we have found it easier to understand when cancer is termed *noninvasive (contained)* or *invasive (noncontained)*. Noninvasive cancer generally means that the atypical cells are still localized in the area where they first started to grow. The bad cells may be pressed against other healthy tissue, but so far they have not invaded beyond their localized site of origin. Invasive cancer has begun the breakthrough into healthy tissue and may or may not have spread to regional or distant sites. The very nature of the disease gives radiologists a detailed guide to follow in diagnosing cancer. If the X ray shows a smooth, rounded, and even-edged object, it is anticipated to be *fibrocystic disease,* a benign change in the breast tissue that is either a cyst or a solid growth that is not life-threatening. If it is uneven, jagged, and irregular on the borders, then cancer is anticipated.

If it has spread, the cancer is said to have *metastasized.* As a rule, the first site it hits is the lymphatic system, which is a part of the body's immune system. There is nothing unusual about cancer spreading to the lymph nodes because these are the disease fighters that trap invaders and kill them. (You have probably experienced swelling under your jaw or under your arm when you've had a particularly bad infection. That was the lymph node at work.)

Unfortunately, the rapidly growing cancer cells sometimes overwhelm the lymph nodes and break loose, spreading throughout the lymphatic network and causing what is called *distant metastases.* This is the spread of cancer to parts of the body other than the breasts. Sometimes the blood acts as the transport system, carrying cancer cells to new sites.

In the case of early detection of the disease, surgery is the treatment of choice for certain cancers. The offending tumor is simply cut out and the patient is sent home, but must return for periodic checkups. The success rate of surgical removal of noninvasive tumors without lymph-node involvement is so good that, in some instances, doctors actually use the word "cure" or assure their patients that they are a hundred percent cancer-free.

There is a debate in the medical community concerning the very nature of cancer. The generally accepted (or public perception) is that noninvasive cancer has remained at the site and apparently no cancer cells have been flushed through the body or there would be lymph-node involvement. Thus the chance of distant metastases is dramatically less. On the other hand, some doctors believe that cancer begins to immediately shed cells that travel throughout the body virtually from day one. In this case, the lymph nodes apparently do their job and kill the cells or the cancer cells are flushed out of the body before establishing a tumor or overwhelming a lymph node. But it matters not which theory your doctor believes because the majority of doctors still arrive at the same conclusion in treatment: A tumor needs to be removed if possible; lymph-node involvement or metastases demands chemotherapy or radiation; or treatment will involve all of the above.

TREATING CANCER

It is extremely important to become acquainted with a few definitions pertaining to the three basic types of cancer treatments. The objective of all of these procedures is to remove not only the *known* cancer cells, but also the unseen and often undetected cancer cells.

Surgery

Surgery is just what the term implies: the surgical removal of the diseased tumor or site. It is performed in a hospital under general anesthesia.

The simplest form of surgery is the *lumpectomy* in which the offending lump is taken out along with a portion of the surrounding healthy tissue. Sometimes a portion of the breast may also be removed. In most cases, the lumpectomy is followed by radiation treatment. Often a few lymph nodes are removed to see if the cancer has spread.

Mastectomy is the surgical removal of the breast and is often the procedure of choice, although earlier detection is beginning to allow surgeons to perform more and more lumpectomies.

There are three types of mastectomies. A *complete* (or simple) *mastectomy* is the removal of the breast only, leaving a scar along the chest wall. It has a flattening effect. Doctors may also elect to take out a few lymph nodes found in that area.

A *modified radical mastectomy* is the removal of the breast, the pectoralis minor muscle, and lymph nodes under the arm in the axillary (armpit) area. This creates a slightly sunken area on the chest wall. Tissue will be cut away from under the arm, depending on the amount of lymph-node involvement.

A *radical mastectomy,* popular until only a few years ago, is now seldom performed. It requires the additional removal of the pectoralis major muscle and is the most disfiguring of all, leaving only a thin layer of skin on the chest wall while limiting mobility in the arms.

The key to which type of surgery is needed, and its success rate, is the stage of the cancer. If the disease is noninvasive, normally the patient's prognosis is outstanding, better than ninety percent. If it is invasive, then each case depends upon the extent to which the cancer has spread to the lymphatic system and to other parts of the body.

Radiation

Radiation treatment calls for the affected area to be bathed with radiation, either before or after the surgery. This is done with pinpoint accuracy and often treatment will call for applications to lymph nodes near affected areas such as the chest, throat, and back. This treatment is conducted in specially shielded rooms, utilizing large machines to kill both known and unknown cancer cells. Sometimes the patient suffers burns. Unless doctors advise hospitalization, the patient can remain at home and visit the clinic daily.

Because of the size of the machinery and the justified fear of radiation, the exacting nature of this treatment is often misunderstood. As with any cancer treatment, there is danger; but every precaution is taken to reduce the threat of overexposure to harmful radiation.

A patient is first taken to a simulator where technicians set up the treatment plan. The size of the tumor is measured, the location is charted, and, finally, the machine is carefully aimed at treatment areas. A special shield is designed to cover the patient so that only the area needing treatment is exposed to the powerful invisible beam. The doctor does not aim the machine and simply fire away. In an effort to minimize the effects of radiation, the tumor is attacked from a number of angles, sparing normal tissue from concentrated exposure while allowing the tumor to receive full exposure from several converging angles. This is why precise measurements are taken.

Finally, the area to be treated is carefully outlined on the patient. Many patients hate these marks, which often extend beyond clothing. These marks are used every day as the patient comes in for treatment. They *do* wear off eventually. Don't be alarmed if the marks indicate that radiation will also be delivered to the armpit, neck, and breastbone. The doctor is irradiating lymph nodes in that area.

When treatment starts, the cobalt beam destroys the cancer cells and the body sloughs off the dead cancer cells internally through the kidneys and bowel, the body's elimination system. The radiation causes a decrease in white blood cells and the patient can experience weakness, mild nausea, and general malaise.

Bob: Jean Neff, a dear friend who had successfully survived breast cancer and had taken radiation treatments, took Martha to her first radiation session.

The technicians measured Martha's body, pinpointed the exact spot for radiation, and meticulously marked the spot with a staining dye that left red guidelines on her cheek, neck, chest, and back.

It was an especially nervous time and Martha was filled with questions.

"Won't the radiation cause me to have more cancer?" she asked the doctor.

"Won't it get all over my body?" was her next concern.

"Each of the beams will pinpoint the exact spot to be treated. A shield will be made to direct it exactly there and protect other parts of your body," he explained.

"It's a lonely feeling," Martha said, treatment after treatment. It was also scary to have shields put around parts of your body, screens erected, and technicians step out of the room as the cobalt bombards you.

"I wanted to get out of there too," Martha explained. "But after the first few treatments, I had learned 'the procedure' and wasn't as nervous."

This doctor was the only one who believed that the cancer could be killed. But even his optimism in those early days of treatment was threatened by an incident within a week of Martha's first visit. The first of three massive doses of chemotherapy had had drastic results, reducing the tumor in her breast and under her arm from near lemon-size to about grape-size. Everyone was excited about the swift decrease.

"You don't know how lucky you are," our family physician told me. "It's terrible to keep giving treatment and all the tumor does is grow, no matter what you do."

About two weeks into the radiation treatment, Martha told me the lump was bigger than it had been. When she told the doctor, he was skeptical; but, ever careful, he decided to remeasure the size of the lump.

To his amazement, it had started to grow again.

He immediately conferred with Martha's oncologist, who put her back on oral chemotherapy. This heightened Martha's radiation burns. But the radiation—coupled with chemotherapy—had a dramatic effect and within weeks the cancer was gone, just as he had predicted.

Since the side effects of chemotherapy are similar to those of radiation, the two are seldom given at the same time, although doctors occasionally are forced to. Chemotherapy tends to heighten the effect of radiation and cause burns. Yes, Martha got burned and spent several restless days on pain medication before the symptoms began to ease. Burns are perhaps the most common side effect of radiation and generally occur toward the end of lengthy treatments. Liquid medication is used to bathe the wounds; medicine in capsule form can help ease the pain. Radiation can also cause general malaise due to a drop in white-blood-cell count. As with chemotherapy, blood samples closely monitor the effects of the treatment.

Chemotherapy

Aside from mastectomy, chemotherapy is perhaps the most feared form of treatment because of its many potential side effects, including severe nausea, hair loss, fatigue, a raw throat, and general malaise. In tailoring your wife's treatment to her specific needs, your doctor can select from a wide assortment of drugs that have been approved for treatment. Based on the type of cancer, location, and stage of development, he may give them singly or in combination. Not all drugs have the same side effects and not all patients experience the same side effects from the same drugs, so we suggest that you reserve judgment until your wife is into her regimen. At best, you can expect it to be difficult for her.

Chemotherapy is the treatment of cancer with powerful drugs designed to kill rapidly multiplying cells. It can be given intravenously through an IV (directly into a vein) or by mouth in the form of tablets. Unfortunately researchers have been unable to program the drugs to kill only the cancer; they also kill good cells. The whole body is affected by the effort to destroy the cancer cells that may have broken away from the primary site. The chemicals attack the rapidly growing normal cells found in your hair, bone marrow, stomach and intestine, and in the lining of the mouth.

The drugs are generally administered by IV in the doctor's office, after which the patient goes home. Some patients react so violently to the drugs, however, that a hospital stay is required. Martha was hospitalized for each of her three major chemotherapy treatments administered over a year's time, while Ann was able to continue working throughout her four-and-one-half-month ordeal.

Your Treatment Options
The doctor is likely to present several choices in two rather broad-based areas:

1. If the cancer is noninvasive, the options could include a lumpectomy or a simple mastectomy. Sometimes, in the presence of several malignant tumors, a simple mastectomy is dictated to remove the chance of other tumors appearing. Depending on the circumstances, the surgery could be followed by radiation or chemotherapy.

2. If the cancer is invasive, the type of surgery will be dictated by the size of the tumor and the degree to which the

disease has spread. Generally, a modified radical mastectomy is needed to remove the tumor from the breast and the axillary (armpit) lymph nodes are removed to see if they are involved; the doctor may have already determined lymph-node involvement based on swelling in the area and X-ray results. Sometimes surgery is needed to remove the cancer from the metastasis site. These procedures are usually followed by either chemotherapy or radiation or both, with the order of treatment determined by site and size. Sometimes radiation or chemotherapy precedes the surgery.

There is an ongoing debate among surgeons, oncologists (cancer specialists), and researchers. Some believe that a lumpectomy, followed by radiation and chemotherapy, is sufficient to treat the disease, thereby saving the breast. Others argue that once the disease has appeared, a woman lives with the constant threat of it returning and the offending site (i.e., the entire breast) should be removed. Sometimes the cancerous tumor is so large (as in Martha's case) that it cannot be removed surgically until radiation or chemotherapy has been used to reduce its size. Sometimes the treatments cause the cancer to disappear. More often than not, the tumor simply reduces in size and the patient then has the opportunity of allowing the doctor to perform a mastectomy.

We stress that the treatment your wife receives will depend on her status at the cancer's discovery. She may undergo all three—surgery, radiation, and chemotherapy.

Ann had a biopsy, followed by a double mastectomy and voluntary chemotherapy. Martha had a biopsy, the first of three major doses of chemotherapy, radiation treatment, two more rounds of chemotherapy, a modified radical mastectomy of the left breast followed by oral chemo, and, finally, a voluntary simple mastectomy.

Each case is different.

Bob: *Martha had little choice in her treatment. The tumor in her breast had metastasized to her lymph nodes under her arm, where it was lemon-size, and the doctor elected to leave* *both virtually untouched when he performed the biopsy. To do otherwise could have caused the cancer to spread.*

A complete plan of action couldn't be mapped out until a series of scans could be made of Martha's liver, spleen, and bones. Blood tests were also being processed to determine if any other cancers—large and unseen—were present. Since cancer had been found in the lymph nodes, there was a real danger that it had already spread to other parts of her body. Until the doctors had some idea of what was going on, there was nothing we could do but wait.

Martha was up and into X ray at six o'clock the morning following the biopsy. Within an hour, blood tests had been run, the skeletal system had been X-rayed, and the liver and spleen had been checked.

We were startled when less than ninety minutes later the doctor burst into the room, grinning from ear to ear. He barely uttered "good morning" before blurting out the good news. The tests had revealed that Martha's vital organs were clear of any detectable signs of cancer. Of course, that didn't mean that microscopic cancer was not lurking somewhere, but it did offer hope.

The doctor had already decided on a plan of action that included chemotherapy and radiation treatment to reduce the cancer to a size small enough to remove surgically.

"What are my chances now?" Martha wanted to know.

"I'd say they are about the same, but let's wait and see what the chemotherapy does," the doctor replied.

Microscopic lab tests had failed to reveal the exact type of cancer Martha had. Clinical evaluation suggested inflammatory cancer, a particularly virulent form of the disease.

"We're going to treat it as if it were the worst kind and give you the strongest possible dose of chemotherapy," the doctor continued. "Then, we'll hope for the very best."

Within a few hours Martha was administered a strong dose of chemotherapy.

Suddenly, we had gone from depression to the first glimmering of real hope. I looked at her lying in that hospital bed.

*She still had life. On that day I could see her and I could touch
her and I could tell her that I loved her. I knew that we would
fight this battle with all we had. I also knew that from now on,
we would take life one day at a time.*

COPING WITH THE SIDE EFFECTS
OF TREATMENT

Our wives suffered all the indignities that go with chemotherapy. We want to emphasize that you should keep reminding her that chemotherapy side effects are generally temporary,
especially hair loss. We spent a lot of time reassuring Ann and
Martha that we loved them and that their hair would grow
back.

Hair Loss
Of all of the side effects, hair loss is the one that takes the
most emotional toll, and is also the most visible. There is no
easy way for her to remove hair once it has died and starts to
come out in her brush. And when it starts to come out by the
handful, be prepared for an emotional time. Hair will usually
return once the treatments stop. To her delight, Martha's extremely fine, baby-soft hair, which she wrestled with for years,
came back with more body and very curly. She was not too
delighted with the fact that it was much darker than her normal
honey-blond; it was almost black. Both these effects lasted for
about two years before the hair lightened to her more normal
color and again became baby-fine, losing its curl. We have
talked to a number of women whose hair grew back in ringlets,
with more body, and in a darker—sometimes different color—
and stayed that way. As with anything else in this cancer
battle, everything depends on the individual. Some women,
including Martha, grow a natural tinge of silver, sort of a "frost-
ing" effect, which has become the envy of those who pay hundreds to get that look at a beauty parlor.

Ann lost a portion of her hair and was unable to color it
her trademark platinum. Therefore, like thousands of other

women, she was forced to wear a wig. It served to add insult to injury.

"Gee, I lost both my breasts, and now my hair," she once told Andy in frustration.

Martha lost her hair three times over the next twelve months. At first she purchased a couple of wigs, but toward the end of her treatment she used several lightweight turbans. They were less fuss than a wig, especially at home. Wearing a turban was also less jarring on her nerves when she walked by a mirror.

Bob: I found Martha standing in the bathroom staring into the mirror. She wasn't crying. There was a mixture of rage and frustration and hopelessness as she showed me the hairbrush filled with dead hair.

For the past few days, the sheen in her hair had begun to fade and hair finally had started to come out. When the hair loss hit, it did so over a few days, first leaving long strands on her pillow and bath towels, and finally matting because you couldn't brush it; each swipe would pull out big globs.

She had tried to keep her hair as long as she could, but it was time to take it off. It had died at the roots and someone needed to gently remove it from her head.

"You want me to do it?" I asked as I reached for the brush.

"No," she said. "Just let me do it by myself."

I understood, so I left her alone. When she came out, she had a bath towel wrapped around her head. I gently began to unwrap it as tears started down her cheeks.

Even prepared, it was a bit of a shock, because she did look different. I took her face in my hands, then kissed her smack in the middle of her bald head.

"Even bald you're the sexiest thing I've ever seen," I told her as I proceeded to cover her pate with kisses.

It took a few days, but soon she was comfortable enough that she didn't worry about keeping her head covered around me.

But she did have a bit of a problem keeping her head warm after the hair loss.

Hair loss is a very real emotional issue. It's hard for a man to understand because we believe that each man, subconsciously, expects to be bald someday. Also, it is acceptable for men to be bald. Several—such as Yul Brynner and Telly Savalas—found fame and fortune only after shaving their heads. There are jokes about men's bald heads: "God made two kinds of heads. One he was proud of and the other he covered with hair."

Doctors acknowledge that "Will I lose my hair?" is often the first question, "Will it grow back?" the second, and "When?" is the third. When women ask about hair loss, they generally refer to their head hair, but the chemotherapy will also cause them to lose *all* of their body hair.

A woman's hair is often considered her crowning glory. It's an attitude that runs deep in the psyches of women *and* men, and has for ages. Think about it. When you go to identify a woman standing at a distance, how do you describe her? She's the blonde, or the redhead, or the brunette. How do you identify a man? He's short or tall or fat or thin, although sometimes you will refer to him by hair color, too.

It may be best to preplan and purchase the wig before the hair starts to fall out because it's difficult to shop once hair is gone.

Nausea and Vomiting
Martha reacted so intensely to the first dose of chemotherapy that she was forced to go into the hospital for each additional treatment. The first dose came the day after the biopsy.

Bob: I had functioned as a bedpan commando before, but everything I had ever done paled in comparison to what was about to take place that Tuesday afternoon after Martha received her first chemotherapy treatment.

Together, Martha and I have always faced adversity. If she was going to be in the hospital, I scheduled vacation time or we arranged to have the surgery done on a Friday so I could check in with her and nurse her through the weekend. And I always ordered up a cot to sleep on during her hospital stay.

We knew that Martha had a "weak" stomach, but to our surprise she had sailed through the biopsy with a minimum of nausea. Still she was leery as the head oncology nurse at the hospital administered the three carefully prepared chemicals.

"Why do you have to use gloves?" was Martha's first question as the nurse pulled on a pair of rubber gloves to handle the toxic compounds.

"Because the drugs are very potent and it's best not to spill them on your skin," she answered. "Sometimes an oncology nurse is pregnant and she has to be especially careful.

"We know you'll have some side effects, but we don't know yet how you'll react. It depends on the individual. Some people can take this at the doctor's office, go home, be sick a few hours, and be back at the job the next day."

"Not me," Martha predicted. "How long will it take before I feel the effects?" she asked.

"I don't know. It's different with each person," the nurse answered as she got up to leave. "Hopefully, you'll be one of the lucky ones."

Then she handed me a card and said, "If you need me, here's my telephone number."

An hour passed, then two, then three and four. The attendant brought dinner.

"I'm hungry, but I'm afraid to eat," Martha said, eyeing the tray.

"Go ahead," I encouraged. "Nothing's happened," before adding with a shrug, "If it does, I'll take care of it."

Martha ate. We began to think that we had this thing licked. Maybe the scare stories were just that, scare stories.

Then it hit all at once—deep, racking heaves similar to those a drunk has after everything's left his stomach. It wouldn't pass. The doctor gave her strong doses of muscle relaxants but to no avail. She fell into a pattern. She would throw up every seven minutes or so. The heaves would last for a few minutes, then the drugs would take over, virtually knocking her out, and she would slip into a deep sleep, only to be aroused again a few minutes later.

Then a new problem developed. The massive amounts of antinausea drugs caused her blood pressure to dip. She was too far out of it to worry, but I did enough worrying for both of us. It wasn't until a nurse told me that her own blood pressure routinely ran eighty over forty that I relaxed.

It was a long night. Fourteen hours after the nausea hit, Martha finally fell into an undisturbed sleep. It was blissful rest for both of us, and for the nursing staff, a group of fine women whom we would come to know well over the next two years. Based on their care, we asked for their wing of the hospital every time we checked in.

Several days later Martha was released to go home, too weak to stay by herself. My mother and my Aunt Lil took turns coming to San Antonio to keep our household operating.

Meanwhile, within a week of Martha's biopsy and first chemotherapy treatment, Ann entered the hospital for her double mastectomy. The diagnosis had come in the middle of an important project that Ann was determined to finish. She was playing the Red Queen in Irwin Allen's musical miniseries *Alice in Wonderland.* Irwin agreed to keep the part open for her.

Andy: Emotions played a unique role in our lives the morning that the doctor confirmed that Ann had breast cancer. That afternoon, she was scheduled to record a song written by Steve Allen called "Emotions" for the audio track of *Alice in Wonderland.*

If that wasn't bad enough, the lyrics contained the words, "Emotions we'll have till we die." When she reached those words, her voice cracked. Only I knew what the reason was. Ann covered her tracks quickly, looking through the thick, soundproof glass at Steve in the control booth.

"Hey, Steve, you sure wrote a two-boxer here!" she exclaimed, referring to their private system of rating sad songs as those requiring one or two boxes of tissues. My impulse was to go to her, but I fought it back, knowing how badly she wanted to finish her work this day.

I swear I didn't say anything to anyone, but Steve and the audio guys just seemed to have some sort of understanding. They hung in there while Ann flubbed that line on several takes. She has a reputation as "one-take Jillian" but it wouldn't apply that day.

"You'll get it, Ann. No rush. Take your time," Steve encouraged her.

"I'm fine," she said with that little gurgle that only I thought I knew was in her voice; a sound that indicated she had been crying. "Take it from the top."

It was the fifth or sixth take and she reached down deep into her emotional reserves to sing that song to perfection. As the last note faded, the guys applauded, led by that great intuitive Steve Allen, who knew something special had just happened, but not just what.

I was proud, scared, and on the verge of tears as we walked to the car holding hands.

"That lyric is a long way off for you. Don't pay it any more attention!" I told her as I hugged her at the car. "You're not going anywhere."

She had a little cry and we went home.

Ann was back on the set of *Alice in Wonderland* just eleven days after her surgery. A real trouper, she upheld the tradition of "The show must go on." Within a few weeks of surgery, she performed with Bob Hope in Dallas and was back on the set of her television series, "It's a Living."

While working in the series, Ann elected to take "precautionary" chemotherapy. Although the doctors found no lymph-node involvement, they suggested Ann and Andy consider limited chemotherapy as "insurance." It also was a case of no one—Ann and Andy or the doctors—wanting to feel responsible if, for some unknown reason, one cancer cell was lurking somewhere within her body.

It's a tough decision. A case can be made for both sides. With Ann's two separate cancer sites contained and surgically removed (double mastectomy), and with no lymph-node involvement, a good argument could have been made against chemotherapy. An equally strong argument could have been made on the side of caution. It's your choice. Ann and Andy wanted to be as aggressive—and thorough—as possible.

Andy: In the end, it was Ann's decision to take the chemotherapy, with my full support. If only one cancer cell was traveling in the body, looking for a place to land and grow, we wanted it killed. And, we thought the price Ann would have to pay was worth it in the long run. Make your own decision and don't be second-guessed by anyone.

I'm happy that women have choices today because years ago they did not. It was simply a matter of cutting out the known cancer and crossing your fingers and praying for the best! And while prayer is always "in," there are more treatment plans available now.

You have to approach chemotherapy with almost a love-hate feeling. That's the way I viewed it when Annie took that chemical concoction.

I loved it because this junk does kill cancer cells but I hated it because it made her so sick. It's just too bad that it also kills some of the good cells.

The doctor mapped out a regimen of treatment for Ann that would require six months of treatment. The plan called for her to receive chemotherapy for two weeks, then rest a week. The chemo would be administered by injection. She was able to take the chemotherapy in the doctor's office and dash back to work on the television series "It's a Living," where she completed her day's work as the nausea built. By six o'clock she rushed home, ran from the driveway to the bathroom, and was sick for the next twelve to fourteen hours. The chemotherapy took such a toll that she elected to stop treatment after four and a half months.

Andy: Everyone remembers that first night of chemotherapy. Yes, we did go out to eat. It was Italian, and Ann had tomatoes. I know because I saw them again later.

This thing seemed to follow a pattern. She had the injection about four-thirty in the afternoon and five hours later we were thinking, "Hey, Ann still feels okay. This chemo is overrated. No big deal."

Then it hit, a night-long session of holding her, my left arm around her waist to keep her from hitting her head. I'd rub her back with my right hand in circle-type motions going counterclockwise. This seemed to help her get "it" up (whatever "it" was) and my left hand would feel her poor little tummy going through hell.

It took us all to get her through these nights—mom, dad, brother Ben, and myself. On a later chemo night, we were all in the bedroom and Ann got this incredulous look on her face.

"This is crazy. Do you realize that you're just waiting for me to get sick enough to throw up?" she asked with a wry chuckle. We tried to laugh, but it was time and we were off and running. Later we were to see a bit of humor in it all. Most people run in the other direction when someone's about to vomit.

Oddly enough, the first night—although bad enough—was not the worst by a long shot.

The worst night, which I call the "night of the bad blood," came just prior to stopping chemo.

From time to time, Ann would vomit a little blood because her esophagus was raw or her stomach lining would tear from all the throwing up. But this night was different. Nothing was left in her stomach and deep, racking dry heaves had settled in for a long stay. I felt helpless, there was just nothing else I could do. I decided to put a little baby food in her stomach with the hope that it would give her something to toss up and satisfy the "urge." I don't think it worked. I think it just made it worse; but I was in the kitchen getting the baby food when I heard this terrified "Andy!"

The first thing I saw was the blood. Bright, deep, red blood. Ann was on the floor by the toilet with a big towel that used to be white.

"Help me!" she tried to yell, the blood bubbling up to her mouth and running down her cheeks.

God, I was scared. I've seen accidents, the victims of murders, the carnage that one man can do to another, but here was my love, blood dripping from her mouth and begging me to help her.

I tossed the towel, grabbed another, wet part of it, and wiped her mouth and face. I looked into her mouth and saw the blood coming again. I couldn't stop it, so I cleaned her face again. By now it had sort of slowed down.

I dressed her as best I could, all the while reassuring her that everything would be okay. I felt like I didn't have time to call an ambulance, so I carried her to the car and sped off to the hospital but not before calling the doctor to meet us there.

It wasn't as bad as it looked. The esophagus and throat had just had it and had started to bleed. The doctor reassured us that there would be no more hemorrhaging that night and there had not been as much blood loss as it appeared.

That happened in the wee hours of the morning. We were exhausted, but she made it to work the next day.

It was especially difficult for me to keep my peace on the set that particular day. Tempers flare and unkind things are said in any work situation. But when you get a group of creative people together you really set the pot to boiling. We all know that when we are healthy, and someone tries to slip a bad one over on us, it's no big deal. But that day, when all these little things happened, I just wanted to step in and say, "Hey, she's sick. Give her a break."

It was like watching a fragile kitty in a cage as mean folks poked a stick at it. But I kept my mouth shut because that's what Ann wanted. She didn't want to be treated any differently because she was taking chemotherapy. But I sure would have liked to have said a word or two to the few cast members who had been jealous of Ann's great success and who felt they had to take cheap shots at her.

Martha's other two doses of massive chemotherapy were not administered until after she had received thirty-seven radiation treatments. She also took oral chemo during the radiation treatments, which heightened the effect of the radiation burns.

It took a year to complete her treatments. After the next two rounds of chemotherapy, Martha had her first mastectomy and the doctor put her back on oral chemotherapy until her body rebelled and she could no longer take the medication without endangering her life. A year later, Martha had her second mastectomy as we were beginning to write this book.

Bob: The next two treatments were no easier. Martha's oncologist just shook his head and admitted that he had never seen a patient react so strongly. In spite of his best efforts— and those of several specialists he consulted—Martha's treatments were nightmares. The doctor spent many hours poring over textbooks and research papers and in discussions with colleagues in an effort to find the proper medication to ease Martha's reaction to the drugs.

Her second treatment stands out for three very diverse incidents. After bringing her home from the hospital, she got progressively weaker. Nothing helped. Even the vitamin-rich supplements I pumped down her failed to bring color to her cheeks.

After several days, the oncologist put Martha back in the hospital. In an attempt to relieve the nausea, medicine had been prescribed that would speed up the action of the intestine. Since that didn't seem to help, it was decided to go in the opposite direction—to slow down the intestine. It worked and within six hours she experienced relief.

Martha was wan, exhausted, and dropped into a light sleep. I called our son and he told me that Hal Wingo of People *magazine had telephoned. The magazine was ready for me to write a cover story on Ann's battle with breast cancer. We had been discussing the project for several weeks and the project had come to fruition at this particularly bad time. Martha encouraged me to leave her in the hospital, go to Los Angeles, and write the story. Ann and Andy were willing to wait, but I felt the story was too important to run the risk of losing a cover on such a popular magazine. While we all believed that the story would save lives, there was no way I would leave Martha, no matter how much she insisted.*

"If all I have in me is one People *magazine cover, then it doesn't make any difference if I write it or not. If I have more than one, then I'll get my shot at it," I assured her, my heart bursting with pride at the good fortune of marrying such a special woman while at the same time feeling like a quarterback just pulled from starting in the Super Bowl.* People *arranged for another writer, John Stark, to help Ann tell her story and, based on the response, it did save lives. The cover story on Ann Jillian turned out to be one of the magazines biggest selling issues of the year.*

A few days later, Martha and I were even happier that I didn't leave. It was a Saturday night and I had fixed her a bed in the living room to give her a change of scenery after bringing her home from the hospital. Her nausea had been pretty bad, so I was bathing her face with a washcloth when I noticed that one side of her mouth sagged downward, giving her a sardonic grin. I watched her for about thirty minutes and it got progressively worse. I was fearful that she was having a stroke. Trying to be casual, I started bathing her face and asking questions I hoped were not too obvious:

"Are you feeling better now?" I began.

"A little," she said.

I stroked the affected side of her face.

"Does that feel good?" I asked.

"Yes," she answered.

"Do you feel funny?" I continued. "Tingle anywhere or anything?"

"No, why?" I could hear her alarm.

"Just curious. You've had so many things happen to you, I just wanted to check you out."

"Does your face feel funny?" I persisted.

"No."

"Why don't you move your legs over here and I'll rearrange the cover and give you a foot massage," I asked, wanting to see if she could still move her limbs. She could and in moving, she also used both arms.

Still confused and concerned, I made an excuse and slipped off to call the oncologist. He knew exactly what was happening. Her body was protesting its prolonged exposure to an antinausea drug. Even though she had several signs of someone having a stroke, the doctor quickly reassured me, although he pointed out the symptoms would last a few hours after we discontinued the dosage.

I decided the best thing to do was tell Martha what was going on. I didn't want her to walk by a mirror and be shocked. She took the news like a trouper, even asking me to bring a mirror so she could look at what the medicine was doing.

The best way to fight the terrible side effects of chemotherapy—aside from medication—is to maintain a positive attitude.

"Remember when we were kids? It always seemed like the best medicine was the worst-tasting," Martha said with a grin.

With each dose or each crisis, I kept reminding her—and myself—that the chemo effects would pass and with them the threat of cancer. We fixed our eyes on the goal of remission. The desire to live can overcome a lot of obstacles.

While nothing we did to ease the effects of chemotherapy worked completely, there were a couple of solutions we arrived at by trial and error that helped in her case; one was mental and the other physical, and often, we combined them.

I had read somewhere that positive thoughts of pleasant places often helped shove aside the continuous queasy feeling in the pit of the stomach; especially if you thought of a safe place where there had been joy and contentment. So, Martha and I spent many hours reliving the glorious wonderful moments of our lives. Often we concentrated on special events, attempting to recall them in detail—who was there, what day of the week, what we wore, what we ate, etc.—or favorite vacations.

But it was the "safe spot" that brought special relief. I had also read that it helped a person to relax by picking a safe spot, somewhere that life is sweet and content and far removed from daily cares.

For me it was a small alcove on the second-floor mezza-

nine of the Contemporary Hotel at Disney World. From there you could look out over the lagoon and watch fellow travelers enjoy the peaceful Florida countryside during the daytime or see a parade of barges gaily decorated with thousands of colored electric lights at night. There, in the middle of that Magic Kingdom, my world was secure and safe, my mate by my side. Many times I transported her there by memory and once we even visited that spot during chemotherapy.

Martha's spot was the beach—any beach she had visited. She liked to recall the hot baking sun, the cool touch of the water, the slippery feel of suntan lotion, the day-long feast of sandwiches and fruit and the peace of mind all these activities brought.

"There is a calming, soothing influence," she said of the water gently breaking on the shore. We would talk about the beach for hours, describing details, beginning sentences with "Do you remember . . . ?"

Often relief came in a simple foot massage. No, I'm no expert on reflexology nor have I ever read a book about it. I just know that one day I briskly massaged her feet and for some reason it helped ease the nausea. Some days it virtually eliminated the sick feelings, other days it had only a limited effect. But it always worked somewhat.

We seemed to have the best results when we combined a foot massage with mental exercises in recalling a favorite event or in whisking our minds away to our safe spot. We spent hours doing this.

Martha has often told me that her greatest fear now is not cancer, but having to go through the agony of chemotherapy again.

Decreased White Blood Cell Count

While chemotherapy is killing the cancer cells, it is also taking its toll on the white blood cells, the ones that kill infection-causing germs. Therefore your wife's body is going through a traumatic transition in which the bad cells die at the expense of the good. The most drastic drop in white cells occurs around seven to fourteen days after treatment and then the good guys begin to build up again after a few weeks. That's why the doctor takes blood each session, to monitor the life cycle of the white blood cells. If they drop too low, he or she may elect to discontinue treatment for a brief period while they rebuild.

So, here are a few commonsense rules we suggest you follow to protect your wife once she has had chemotherapy and her decrease in white blood cells has put her at risk for infection.

1. Naturally, avoid anyone with infections, colds, or other contagious diseases. A simple case of the sniffles for someone else or a routine childhood disease could be extremely rough on your wife. If you have small children in your home, this will require the utmost delicacy. They want to see their mother. Check with the doctor. Maybe they can wear a surgical mask.

2. You probably already do, but wash your hands before preparing her meals, after using the bathroom, and before changing any of her surgical dressings. That's basic hygiene, anyway.

3. Try to avoid cuts or breaks in her skin. Make sure she wears sturdy shoes and that she protects her hands from cuts and burns by pulling on a pair of gloves when she performs simple chores like washing dishes or working in the garden. Promptly wash any cuts with soap and water and bandage, if necessary.

4. Let her get a little sun, but avoid sunburn.

5. Do not let her take any medication or drink any alcoholic beverage unless approved by your doctor. Some medications may nullify the chemotherapy or hamper its reaction. She should avoid any vaccines as well as persons who have recently been vaccinated against mumps, measles, polio, or smallpox.

6. Watch her for any sign of infection, such as a fever that lasts for more than four hours, burning or frequent urination, itching in the genital area (or anywhere for that matter), and any changes in the skin, such as redness, swelling, tenderness, discharge, or drainage.

7. Practice proper oral hygiene. The anticancer drugs may affect the tender lining of her mouth. Follow several precautions. Have her rinse her mouth every three or four hours with a prescribed mouthwash; if her gums are bleeding, have her brush with a baby-soft toothbrush or a piece of wet gauze or Q-tip to keep them from bruising; keep her lips moist with Vaseline; and avoid spicy foods. Mouth ulcers may develop anyway.

Does this mean you're going to make a hermit out of your wife? Of course not. Martha went on trips to the grocery store and to church while Ann continued to work on her television series. We are just urging a little caution. You know what they say about an ounce of prevention.

As Ann went back to work and began her campaign to help others, Martha faced one of her greatest pleasures and one of her most painful decisions. She had always wanted to go to Hawaii and, as a special treat and incentive, Bob offered to take her there. The day of her chemotherapy treatment, Bob put Hawaii travel posters in her hospital room and circled the departure date—eleven days away—on a calendar. Martha staggered to her feet and made the deadline. The day before they left, she went by the doctor's office to be checked.

Bob: *"You'd better think about having both breasts removed," Martha's oncologist said.*

We were flabbergasted. The radiation and chemotherapy had been so successful that there was no sign of cancer. There had even been hints that no surgery would be required at all.

We also found ourselves in the middle of a medical controversy. The oncologist wanted to be careful, that's why he recommended that both breasts be removed. The surgeon thought that one breast should go but not two.

But in the end, it was Martha's decision.

"You could have a doctor come in and examine you, and if he didn't know your history, he'd swear you didn't have breast cancer, or ever had it," the surgeon explained to her. "But we don't know if there is cancer there microscopically. Just one cell left from the inflammation could cause cancer, just one cell in the top of your skin."

Needless to say this weighed on our minds during the "dream" trip.

"I have to be dying to get to go to Hawaii," was Martha's rueful observation.

"I could be talked out of any surgery" each of the doctors had told her. So, when we returned from our trip, it was second, second-opinion time. A panel of experts from the University of Texas Health Science Center checked her and one doctor advised giving her another (fourth) dose of massive chemotherapy. (Martha had gone as far as she could go. We felt a fourth dose of chemotherapy would have done her in. And the oncologist didn't believe it was necessary.) These experts also gave worse odds than the oncologist, one even going so far as to give Martha only a twenty percent chance of survival, even though the cancer had disappeared. But all agreed that the mastectomy would be proper procedure.

Next we visited our radiologist, who also felt that surgery was the safest approach.

It was decision time, so we took a pen and paper and made a list of reasons why Martha should have surgery and why she shouldn't with the words "We could be talked out of it" echoing in our minds.

Try as we could, the only argument we could muster against surgery was "cosmetics." We felt the pain of surgery and discomfort of treatment did not deserve consideration since she was healthy enough to make it through the postoperative ordeal.

But we had impressive reasons in favor of the surgery.

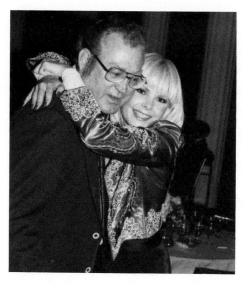

Ann Jillian and Bob Stewart on the night they met, in June 1981. *(Martha Stewart)*

Ann and Andy enjoy their favorite hobby during the good times prior to their battle with breast cancer. *(Hal Uchida)*

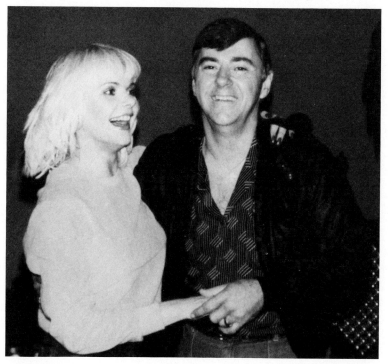

Ann works out in her studio to
get back in shape after
surgery. (Andy Murcia)

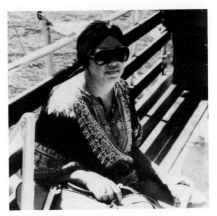

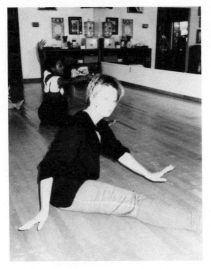

Martha used a black turban to
good advantage on a Hawaiian
cruise. (Bob Stewart)

Ann works out in her studio to get
ready for filming The Ann Jillian
Story. (Andy Murcia)

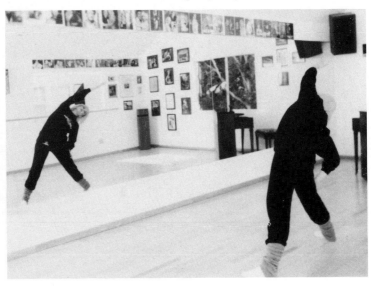

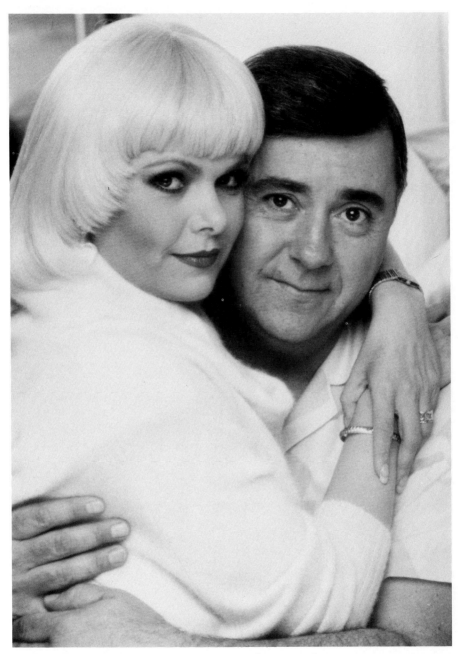

Ann and Andy enjoy a private moment in this 1985 photo.
(Wayne Williams)

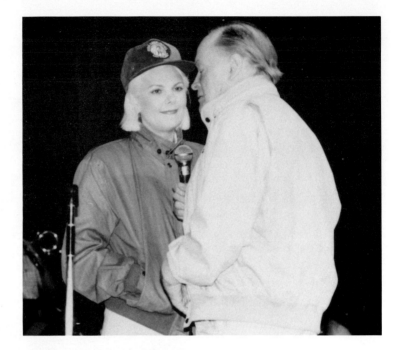

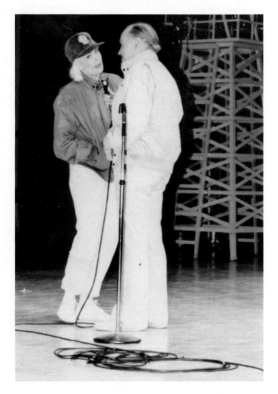

Ann in rehearsal with Bob
Hope for their Dallas, Texas,
performance. *(Andy Murcia)*

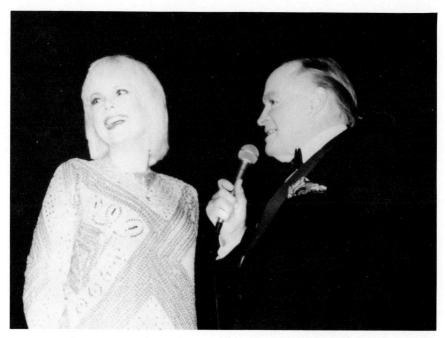

Ann in performance at the Dallas, Texas, Bob Hope Special.

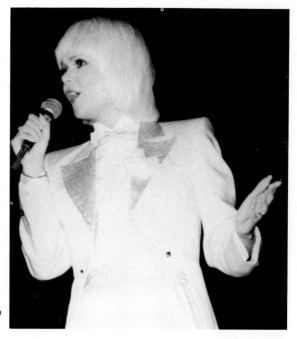

Ann in a club
performance.

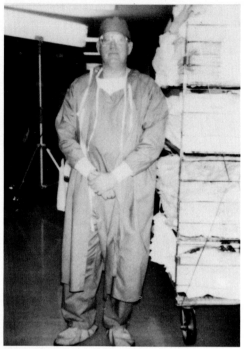

Bob dresses in surgery uniform
for his role (as guerney aide)
in *The Ann Jillian Story.*

Andy (left) and Bob (right) working on the manuscript for
Man to Man.   *(Bobby Stewart)*

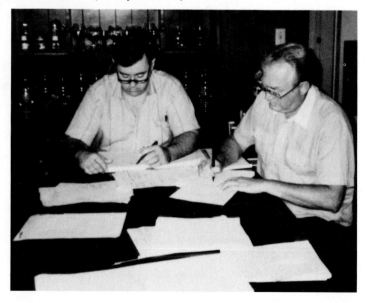

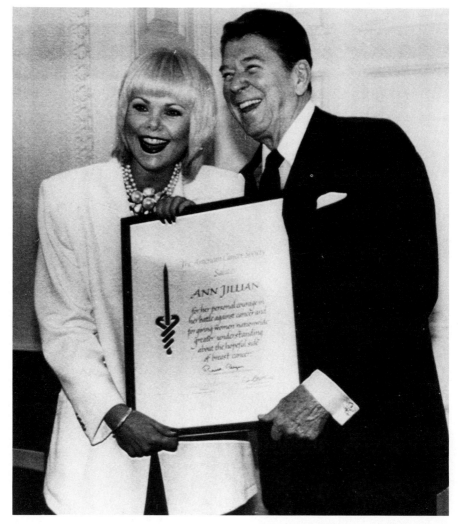

Ann receives the 1986 American Cancer Society Courage Award from President Ronald Reagan on March 20, 1986. *(AP/Wide World Photos)*

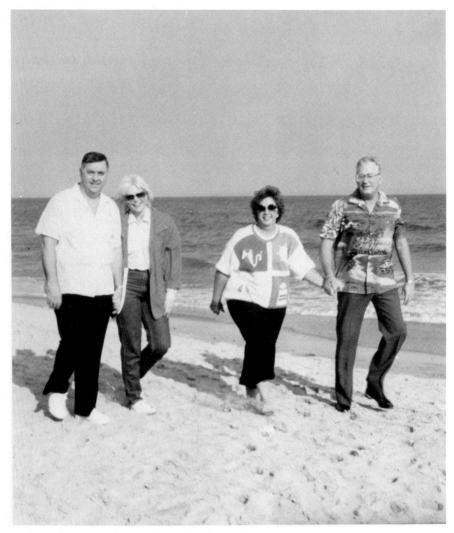

Andy and Ann with Martha and Bob on the beach at Atlantic City.
(Suzanne Opton)

1. It could be life-saving. If cancer cells were present in the primary site, then they would be removed by a mastectomy.

2. Peace of mind. The same reason as above, plus, a mastectomy was the only way to be "one hundred percent sure" that the treatment had been successful and the cancer was gone. The doctors explained that the amputated breast would be extensively checked in the hospital laboratory.

3. A chance to continue our lives together, to grow old together. Would it not be better to be missing a breast, even two, than the whole person?

4. A lack of vanity. We were down to brass tacks and the real issue was life, not cosmetics.

(A year later we added a fifth reason to the list when Martha faced a decision concerning a second mastectomy: 5. No backache! Ever since the first mastectomy, Martha suffered discomfort from backache; some days it was worse than others, but it was always a nagging problem. The breast that had been removed was heavy, and following surgery, her body was out of balance. Even a heavy prosthesis failed to correct, much less ease, the problem. Don't jump to the wrong conclusion. Martha didn't have a mastectomy just to keep her back from hurting. But in light of the first surgery, and the present circumstances, the desire for relief was factored into our decision on the second mastectomy. And, yes, her back quit hurting following the second mastectomy.)

We still have this original list, and drag it out occasionally, should we begin to question our judgment.

I was very vocal in support of the first mastectomy. The loss of a breast seemed a small price to pay for the peace of mind it would give Martha. (When I say small price, I realize the sacrifice, but the issue here is life.*) And, in the end, peace of mind was our prime motive. We reasoned that should cancer be discovered in the lab tests, then Martha had done the right thing, the breast had to go; she surely didn't want it. If the primary sites in her breast and lymph nodes were clear, then* *we knew that she was on the road to recovery and a sacrifice had to be made for both knowledge and peace of mind. Furthermore, we would take that to mean that the chemotherapy and radiation had also had the same effect on any cancer cells that may have left the primary site.*

She elected to have the first mastectomy. All the lab tests were negative; nothing was found.

IT'S TIME TO PITCH IN

You're going to have to learn patience. These treatments take time. Both our wives received surgery and chemotherapy over a year's time, which means you may have to learn some new talents and use them over an extended period.

Call your mom, a grandmother, an aunt, a sister, or your wife's best friend because it's time for you to learn how to use a few household items, if you don't know already. During this year, there will be a house to clean, clothes to wash, food to prepare, and hundreds of other domestic details that will need your attention.

Don't fool yourself into thinking the physical battle against cancer means simply caring for your wife's physical needs. She will be too weak to perform many of her routine household chores and that's where you step in. Encourage her to do as much as she can because following a routine can be very therapeutic. But it will be weeks before she is back to normal. It's up to you to keep the household functioning, although she'll probably feel well enough to supervise a cooperative effort by you and the children.

So, tie on an apron. Don't try to do as good a job as she does. Just try to get the job done while keeping one word in mind—clean! Chemotherapy or radiation will have reduced her immunity. She is more susceptible to germs than ever before. Clean should be everyone's watchword. Keep bedclothes fresh, floors swept, carpets vacuumed, bathrooms spotless, and dishes sparkling.

We suggest that you take a few minutes and develop a

schedule, even if you've never done it before. What are your family's needs for the week? Groceries need to be purchased. Meals prepared. Children taken to school. Clothes washed. Make your list then contact the appropriate support person or organization.

If your youngsters are old enough to do chores, assign them work and make sure they follow through. Older children can learn to prepare simple but nutritious meals. Besides, it will do them good to learn to cooperate; in times of trouble, the whole family pulls together.

Evening meals have to be cooked (Bob's family tagged him the king of hamburger helpers), a wash day set aside (Saturdays are good), dishes to wash (a nightly chore), don't forget breakfast (leave the kitchen clean by getting out of bed a few minutes earlier), and lunch needs to be left in the refrigerator for your wife if no one is staying with her.

It will take a little extra effort, but the reward of watching her improve every day will be worth it.

DO I HAVE ANY OTHER CHOICES?

When it comes to your wife's health, nothing is too much to ask. We know that if a doctor had asked us to stack greased bowling balls at a forty-five-degree angle while standing on our head in a bathtub on the wing of an airplane at forty thousand feet while wearing boxing gloves, we would have gladly tried it without a parachute. Desperate times call for desperate measures so don't be surprised if you find yourself questioning conventional treatment after hearing some of the claims of near-miraculous cures made by proponents of alternate treatments. Because of these claims, you may feel almost compelled to investigate some of the better-known alternatives.

We know that both you and your wife will run into friends and acquaintances who insist on telling you about clinics in the Caribbean or Mexico or South America where desperately ill people go to be cured. These stories are terribly tempting. Instead of the often violent chemotherapy and its debilitating results or invasive surgery, which reshapes your body, patients spend pleasant hours in the sun taking a (supposed) healing combination of natural ingredients. Who wouldn't listen twice to such stories; who wouldn't wish this type of cure for his loved one?

But in the literature we have read and in the conversations we have had with alternate-treatment believers, two things become clear.

First: The vast majority of alternate-treatment leaders claim they have the true "cure" for cancer, but that the rest of the world—especially the medical community—is keeping this "cure" a secret.

Second: The treatments are extremely expensive and such treatment centers are generally inconvenient to reach.

We believe the desire—and often the need—to explore these claims is only natural. You want what is best for your wife.

Should you desire to check out alternate treatments, you are going to find yourself on your own. Common sense tells you that the established medical community doesn't approve of these treatments, or it would use them. Therefore, you will be flying in the face of collective, and conventional, medical wisdom.

We are not going to list the dozens of alternate treatments available. We want you to know that someone understands your feelings, should you decide to investigate. We encourage you to study the topic, collect all the information possible, talk to your doctors, talk to someone who has had firsthand experience, and use sound common sense when making your decision.

Be careful, some of these treatments can be dangerous.

Bob and Martha investigated the use of Laetrile, positive-thinking clinics, and special diets. We'd like to point out that, in our cases, our wives chose to remain under standard medical treatment.

7

That First Prosthesis and Reconstruction

Breast prostheses are available in a bewildering variety of shapes, sizes, and colors. Some are lightweight or hollow, others are heavy. Some are made of rubber, others retain heat and are natural to the touch. Some are made for sports (swimmers can purchase a hollow form with holes for drainage) and others are made for daily wear.

Personal choice must shape your decision. There is no right or wrong but only what is pleasing. By now, your wife probably will have had limited exposure to and use of a soft prosthesis brought to her by a knowledgeable volunteer from the American Cancer Society. At the doctor's request, the ACS sends a Reach to Recovery volunteer with a soft prosthesis form with material to mold it to the right shape, and a special, elastic bra with pockets. She helps your wife shape the device to her specifications so that, should your wife elect, she can make the trip home from the hospital wearing the bra and soft prosthesis over her bandages. Of course, the volunteer is open to all questions as she also teaches your wife simple exercises to speed her recovery.

Before your wife goes to purchase a prosthesis, be sure you get a prescription from the surgeon. This prescription is honored by most insurance companies and they will pay a portion of the costs when you submit the prescription with the bill.

You can prepare a list of stores specializing in prostheses by telephoning the ACS. Although the society makes no recommendations, it provides you with general information on the various types of prostheses. *You* have to make the choice; and we suggest you visit several stores before purchasing. You might also ask for information on mail order, although we found that a personal fitting by an expert works best. A good source of information is one of the local self-help groups.

Bob: It occurs to me that women should have another alternative when shopping for a prosthesis. The experts stress that breast cancer is a very personal disease; each woman reacts differently. Yet women are expected to purchase a prosthesis like they do a pair of shoes, by shopping for size and shape. While it's true that most needs can be met though standardized manufacturing, what about the women who have had more radical surgery? The bras tend to slip up into the sunken area of the chest and the prostheses have a tendency to fall away from the chest wall, pulling and dropping forward so as to put undue stress on the back.

It may be more comfortable for women who've had more radical surgery to have a prosthesis shaped to fit their bodies. Of course it would be more expensive, but it's worth the money in some cases. So, suggest that your wife consider that option. Companies who tailor a prosthesis to your wife's body are difficult to locate, but they are out there.

If you can go with her to shop for a prosthesis it may help, but don't feel hurt if she elects to make that shopping trip alone or with another woman, preferably someone who knows the ropes.

When she comes home to show you her new feminine shape, don't dismiss it. Check her out thoroughly and give her an honest evaluation. We believe that a husband's frank, honest approval means more to a woman than all the sidelong glances in the world. Her dress may not hang right. One breast may be higher than the other (a common problem). If a blouse or dress-top does not close properly, you might both search for the right brooch or pin. There can be minor problems that need a husband's helpful touch. This will also involve you in helping her adjust to this new way of life. It may take several sessions to help her settle in, so be patient and helpful! Remember, she needs your frank opinion because she only wants to look her best.

WHAT ABOUT RECONSTRUCTIVE SURGERY?

This is as personal a decision as one can make. Your wife's choices will be dictated by medical factors peculiar to her case. Reconstruction is not something every woman can automatically have. Some women are good candidates while others—due to treatment—cannot even consider the possibility. And bear in mind that reconstruction is more than one surgery; it can involve a series of operations.

We encourage both of you to fully investigate the pros and cons of the issue, and not to be bullied into a decision by anyone.

This is a decision that needs to be discussed—and decided—before surgery so that should you elect reconstructive procedures, the doctor can perform the mastectomy with that in mind. Some physicians will perform the reconstruction while others prefer to call in a specialist—such as a plastic surgeon— to work with him or her on the day of the surgery. Again, your wife's individual case will determine whether the work is started the day of mastectomy or several weeks, maybe months, later. The surgeon and your wife will also determine if implants are to be used or if a section of her back muscle— still attached to its blood supply—is utilized. Various options should be carefully explored before making a decision.

Neither of our wives chose to have reconstruction; with our very strong support, we might add. In our eyes they were still very complete, whole women, even without breasts. But because of our culture's emphasis on breasts—as evinced in films and commercials—deciding against reconstruction can be controversial. If you want to set our wives to sizzling, then mention the public criticism reported in the press and on television of First Lady Nancy Reagan because she elected to have a mastectomy instead of a lumpectomy and then declined to have reconstructive surgery.

"That makes my nostrils flare!" Ann has said of such criticism.

"It's no one else's business but hers," Ann has said. "She did what was right for her, and any judgment made by anyone without complete access to our First Lady's medical records is an ignorant one."

"It is a very personal and private decision that should be made by each wife and husband," Martha added. "They know what is best for them and what they can accept."

We've discussed this topic with several doctors and they all bring up reconstruction in sessions with patients.

"I'm amazed. I encourage them to have it if they want it and, if they don't want it, to forget it," one doctor said before pointing out that there seems "to be some force out there that brings pressure on a woman to have reconstruction.

"Their attitude seems to be 'Am I wrong because I don't want it? Is there something wrong with me?' They feel very insecure about themselves if they don't want reconstruction," he said. "I've never done any scientific research on it and I've never been able to pinpoint what causes that feeling."

Had she desired it, Ann could have had reconstructive surgery and she has occasionally faced criticism of her decision in question-and-answer sessions when she speaks. She chose not to have it because she thought her body had been through enough trauma, having had a double mastectomy, and she did not feel the need to wear her prosthesis inside her body, instead of outside.

Andy: Ann has never talked against reconstruction itself. She has merely stated that she did not choose to have it and that she is a woman who wants all women to have choices. She will

stand up for any woman out there who wants to have reconstruction, but she would also hope that women would also
stand up for her own right not to have reconstruction.

I always felt that whatever Ann wanted in this area was
good enough for me. So, it was really her decision and I agreed
totally with her choice.

———

*Bob: Because of her medical history, I would have
strongly discouraged Martha from having reconstructive surgery. Prior to cancer she had had three major operations. With
the biopsy and mastectomies added to that, her body had suffered enough as far as I was concerned.*

*Although I didn't favor it, I insisted that we talk to the
surgeon about reconstruction, just to help Martha keep her
options open. He said it would be impossible because he'd had
to remove as much tissue as possible because of the inflammatory nature of her cancer.*

*I would have supported her if she had wanted it for emo-
tional and mental health; but I must admit I would have tried
to talk her out of it. The fact that she was alive—and with
me—was more than enough to make up for a couple of scars.
There are many more important considerations, and much
more beauty, in this world than physical attractiveness alone.*

The important thing to remember is that breast reconstruction
is a personal decision. Consult your doctors, talk to other
women who have had the surgery, and carefully consider all
sides of the issue. Do not let the world make either of you feel
guilty for your decision. If you want to have reconstruction,
that's fine. If you don't, then that's fine, too. Remember it is
your wife's decision—with your input and support.

RETURNING TO THE WORLD

Women who have had mastectomies admit that the first
time they step out in public, they believe that all eyes are
trained on them. This, of course, is not so. Unless you are a
public figure, no one knows.

Andy: Ann's return to the public eye was in three stages.
She went to church, she finished a miniseries, and, just six
weeks after surgery, she stepped onstage in Dallas to thunder-
ous applause as the opening act of a black-tie fund-raiser star-
ring Bob Hope.

The telegram came while she was still in the hospital.

"Hey, Annie, get out of the hospital, they're playing our
intro music." It was from Bob Hope and it gave Ann even more
of a reason to fight. Her surgery was April twelfth and the
opening date with Bob was May fifth.

Ann insisted that we keep the date. I know her feelings
about performing in public for the first time since the surgery
were very turbulent but she kept most of them inside. Occasionally she'd mention, "I hope they accept me in time for my
talents and critique me on how I sing or dance or act—good or
bad—and not on if I have breasts or not."

The night of the show Ann was wound tight, prepared for
heaven knows what. José Ferrer was master of ceremonies.
The master actor/director gave Ann a great introduction, pay-
ing homage to her and the tradition of "the show must go on."

The music started for Ann's opening number. As she
walked onstage and started to sing, the ovation was truly
Texas-sized and the audience went wild. Here was this very
rich, very gray-haired crowd acting like Bruce Springsteen
fans. It was wonderful, just like in a movie. They stood up for
my Ann in Texas! Wow!

Ann was in tears. Conductor Nelson Kole attempted to
start the music again, and again the crowd started to applaud.
Again Ann cried and, again, José came out and motioned the
audience to sit down. Finally, Ann was off and singing "With
a Song in My Heart." The audience applauded wildly after each
song, and some forty minutes later she was ending her show
with the dramatic ballad from *Dreamgirls,* "I'm Not Going." At
the end she tried to strike her usual pose, head back, one hand
reaching to the sky, the other pointing downward. Only this
time the "skyward" arm would not make it to her shoulder,
much less the sky. It just barely cleared Ann's waist because

the surgery still hampered her movements. Again there was a standing ovation.

I know I will never forget that first big audience in Dallas and how kindly and lovingly they received her. I think that this very positive and loving experience led the way for her to reenter show business on a positive note, in a most secure way.

Ann had to accept reality immediately and step into the public spotlight, but most women are more fortunate. Their first trips in public after mastectomy are either to church or synagogue, where friends are thrilled to see them, or on a brief shopping jaunt amid strangers.

But that first public appearance can be traumatic because most women react to cancer surgery as if it were an open secret, for all the world to see. She knows that's not so, but she can't help feeling vulnerable, so be sensitive to her fears.

And there's another concern that bears consideration because it can make that secret fear a reality: the shared dressing area. It's one thing to share a dressing area before mastectomy, but it may be another (even with reconstruction) following mastectomy. Shared dressing areas or shared showers in some recreational facilities may strike cold fear in her heart. We know of one woman (who had had reconstruction) who went on a skiing trip only to discover that the only bathing facility was a shared shower. She went ahead and shared the shower, feeling as if all eyes were on her. She said that no one said anything, so she's unsure if her reconstruction was even noticed or if she was just with a group of sensitive people. But can you image the emotional turmoil she experienced in making the courageous decision to share the shower?

So, before either of you becomes trapped by a similar situation, make a plan. If you're off to the beach, she might dress before you leave or you might stop at a service station where a restroom can afford privacy. You will probably run into this problem when participating in most sports. It's not a major inconvenience, but can turn into a major emotional trauma if not handled properly.

8

The Emotional Battle

PUT YOURSELF IN HER SHOES

You and your wife will be buffeted by a wild array of emotions. Fear is the predominant one and it's okay to be fearful. It's a natural state; just don't let your fear paralyze you.

You will also experience tremendous stress, especially at diagnosis, treatment, and test-result time, and while trying to make decisions about treatment.

The shock of the diagnosis will be followed by disbelief. Most women do not even experience the slightest pain before a breast cancer diagnosis. You and your wife may feel anger—at everything and everyone—and, unfortunately, sometimes at each other. Sometimes there is denial, which can be especially dangerous as some couples search until they find a doctor who tells them what they want to hear. You will bargain—generally with God—and finally anxiety and depression will be followed by a measure of acceptance, by both you and your wife.

Dealing with this emotional storm is unlike any physical battle where you can see and touch and confront your adversary head on. You are now on the threshold of a shadow world where your wife will privately confront her darkest fears and deepest anguish. It will require all your tact, skill, and sensitivity to allow her to open up and invite you into this world. Sometimes the most innocent question, a simple nod of your head, or a casual word can unleash torrents of clashing emotions. You will need to learn to play the game with a poker face. In her precarious state, physical suffering and mental anguish can combine to make a problem seem almost insurmountable.

We live in a society that puts great emphasis on female breasts. Her problem is twofold: her fear of dying is compounded by her dread of losing the symbol of her feminity and female sexuality. So, we challenge you to take a few minutes and reflect on your wife's dilemma. Be frank with yourself as you consider her emotional state. As fearful and confused as you may be, those emotions are undoubtedly ten thousandfold stronger in your wife. As best as you can, try to project yourself into her situation. She faces not only the possibility of death, but also the partial loss of her physical sexuality through mastectomy. And while you are coping with the situation and being supportive—which should ease her fears on this score—believe us, she will be deeply concerned that she could lose her sex appeal for you, her husband—even though you have pledged your eternal love.

Andy: The night before Ann's surgery was one of the longest I've ever lived. When we were getting ready to go to bed, Ann was in the bathroom for quite a while. I became worried and went to the door, which was open a bit.

I looked in and saw my wife cupping her breasts while staring at herself in the bathroom mirror. Silent tears were running down her face and onto her breasts. Her mouth was in the crying position, but she was completely quiet, trying not to let me hear her in her agony.

I opened the door and stood behind her. Ann began to cry aloud as I put my arms around her. We faced the mirrors, both of us crying, my arms folded across her chest, holding her hands.

"I was coming out of the shower and I caught sight of myself in the mirror and realized that this was one of the last

times I would ever see my breasts. It depressed me and I started crying and I didn't want to disturb you."

I reassured Ann that I always wanted to share her thoughts and emotions. Then indicating her very beautiful breasts, I said: "It's hard to fathom, babe, but we must realize that those breasts are like two loaded thirty-eight–caliber pistols aimed right at your heart. They were going to try to kill you, but thank heaven we caught them at it. They must go, so we can save your life. As much as I once loved them, I now hate them with a passion and want them gone so the cancer in them won't kill you."

I had already lost my wonderful mother, Rose, and my loving sister, Dolly, to cancer. Mom died with a lump the size of an orange in her breast. Dolly died of lung cancer. Like so many others whose lives have been affected by cancer, I associated death with the disease. I had to learn that in many cases there is life after cancer, especially if the cancer is detected and dealt with early.

That night, before I had learned my lesson about life after cancer, Ann and I held each other for hours and cried our eyes out. At one point we were kneeling on the bed, just hugging each other, trembling; first Ann and then me, each trying to comfort the other. Both of us would try to think of something to say that would shake us out of this terrible time of fear and help us to sleep. At least asleep, we could avoid the pain in our hearts and let our poor minds rest.

But sleep did not come easy that night and before it did, two very scared people, who felt all alone in the world, had but one place to turn for strength and peace. It was to God. We prayed out loud, together, and sleep came soon after.

We were both fortunate in the way our friends rallied to our side and we say, turn unashamedly to yours. Often people turn inward at a time of trial, but we believe this challenge can best be met by asking for and accepting help from your friends.

Bob had more than twenty friends and family with him when Martha had her biopsy. For a week, one friend would come to the hospital early in the morning and sit in the second-floor waiting room until late each evening as Martha suffered through those early days of chemotherapy. "I'm here to fetch and carry," she told Bob. "You just come get me when you want something."

Andy: Several weeks before we found out that Ann would need surgery, we had a nice visit with a pair of old friends who'd shared the tough times when Ann was trying to launch her career.

When it was decided that Ann would need round-the-clock nursing care, I turned to them as we faced the most difficult challenge of our lives. We'll call them Eddie and Jean to protect their privacy, but we wanted the world to know their role in Ann's recovery. They had just used up all their vacation time to visit us, and it didn't seem possible for Jean to take additional leave.

"Give us an hour and we'll be back in touch," they said.

I knew that we would be able to hire excellent nursing help for Ann, but it just wouldn't be the same without Jean supervising her care. It was something Ann and I wanted very much.

True to their promise, the phone rang a short while later.

"We got it covered. Both of us will be there! Jean will take care of Ann and I will take care of you, buddy."

Our two great friends had switched their work schedules and pulled off the near-impossible.

When Ann was wheeled into her room a few hours after surgery, Jean was standing there, calm, collected, and in charge, just like she always was when running the emergency room at a major hospital in New York. What Ann didn't know is that just minutes before, Jean had been running down the hospital's halls with luggage in hand, having just stepped out of a limo from the airport.

As we anticipated, our friend Jean was able to mix friend-ship and a professional attitude to help guide Ann through this ordeal. She was not the least bit impressed by the Ann who was on TV and all that star stuff. Jean is a tough Irish nurse who runs the ER overnight shift at a hospital near a high-crime area in New York City. Knife and gunshot wounds are common occurrences. Nothing much could get to her.

Jean provided a strong shoulder to lean on, and her professional expertise enabled her to answer Ann's steady stream of questions. Ann's biggest concern at this stage was what type of cancer she had and whether or not the cancer had spread to the lymph nodes and beyond. (A few days later, the lab report would put all those fears to rest with the report that no lymph nodes were involved.)

Jean was also there when Ann wanted to discuss me; specifically, how I would react to having a wife without breasts. Ann was really able to open up and discuss her concerns, without having to worry about upsetting me or her parents.

In addition to her nursing duties, Jean played an important role in keeping the suite secure from press and photographers. I had heard that the tabloids had put out a "feeler" for a photograph of Ann while she slept in her hospital bed. Apparently, they wanted to put it on the cover as a "first photo" after surgery. The topper is I heard they offered twenty-five thousand for the picture. I've known people to do a lot of things for twenty-five dollars, much less twenty-five thousand.

With Jean on duty I could rest a lot easier at home at night.

THE GREAT UNVEILING

"I've never had a husband meet me at the waiting-room door to ask me what his wife looks like after a mastectomy," a doctor once told us. Since we've been in this arena, we can't think of a time we've heard that question either.

The question most often asked is "Is she all right?" And it is now your job to make sure she *is* all right and to help her overcome any difficulties she may have because of surgery. It is unfortunate that a mastectomy is sometimes called "mutilation." That's not a very pretty word and as Martha has said, "It hurts to hear it used." Bob tends to call Martha's scars "beauty marks." To him they're beautiful because without them, he would not have the love of his life.

Bob: *I didn't want Martha to have to wrestle with the problem of the "great unveiling," so I determined to be present when the bandages were first removed.*

We had been through several surgeries, but this time it was different—for both of us. The surgeon clapped his hands together and began rubbing them, as he always did to warm them before examining her. It had been three days since the surgery as he began to peel off the large mound of bandages, which, until now, had given Martha the appearance of retaining her breast.

Martha was apprehensive. I set my face in stone.

"If you've ever had to control yourself, now is the time," I warned myself. "Don't flicker an eyelash."

I was afraid to let any emotion show lest it be misread. Martha had already used the term "mutilation" in describing the surgery. And even though I had reassured her of my love and knew she was secure in that respect, what was about to happen would try even the most secure person.

Martha kept looking down at her left side as the final bandage was removed. Sure the breast was missing, but we had already reasoned that that was the price we had to pay for peace of mind. Test reports following surgery had confirmed that there was no cancer in the breast and I was concerned that Martha would now be sorry that she had elected the surgery. She had been in a unique situation. After chemotherapy and radiation, the doctors had said that they no longer could detect cancer.

But there was still a nagging doubt. Had the chemotherapy and the radiation gotten it all? Were any cancer cells, even a single one, still left in the breast or in the outer layer of skin? There was only one way to be certain and that was to have the mastectomy.

In my mind, Martha couldn't lose. But now, as the bandages came off, I was concerned that she would lose her resolve.

Would she still be pleased with her sacrifice to achieve peace of mind? Would she resent the fact that I pushed for surgery?

All this flashed through my mind as I looked at the results of the doctor's work. The tightly stitched incision started in the left center of her chest and made a gentle spiral upward under Martha's arm, where the more radical surgery had been performed. In an effort to remove the offending lymph nodes, the doctor had cored the armpit. The majority of her skin had been neatly cut away and what little remained had been pulled taut across her ribs and gathered at the incision, where each stitch caused it to pucker. A drainage tube led from the bottom of the incision.

"If we didn't put that in, you'd swell up like a toad," the surgeon explained. The tube was attached to a compressed plastic ball that had a suctioning effect, drawing the fluid out from under the incision. "You don't want any fluid to collect there," the doctor said.

He let me empty the drainage container, so I'd know how to do it once we got home.

The surgeon had removed as much outer skin as possible and had pulled the remaining tissue taut.

"All that skin was once red and inflamed. We didn't want to leave any that we could take," he said, examining the chest wall, which now had a slight concave surface. "I had to stretch it rather tight and it might be uncomfortable, but it'll loosen up."

I didn't have to worry about flinching; it wasn't that bad. If either of us was expecting a raw, ugly-looking wound, we were surprised. The skin had already started healing. From that time on, I bathed and dressed the surgical incision.

"That doesn't look so bad," I said, looking Martha in the eyes. She glanced down at the red welt as I drew her attention to it and entered into the conversation.

Scars and "mutilation" were not our concern. **Life** *was our concern and Martha had not only life, but also the promise of a future. I couldn't have loved her more.*

Although you wife's figure has been altered, she is still the same person. But no amount of preparation can ready her for the shock of what her body looks like after surgery. Now is the time to step in with some old-fashioned honesty. Sure she has changed physically, but your love for her remains strong. Reassure her of this. And don't try to act like nothing has happened to her. Credit her with intelligence. Something *has* happened, but it is nothing that changes your love for her. You will adjust with her.

Help her recall those special moments in your life together that have nothing to do with physical beauty. Think about the reasons that a man remains faithful to his wife. Herein lies the beauty of spiritual love, which transcends the physical and has sustained millions of families since time began.

This is the reassurance she needs now and the attitude you need to cultivate. Don't be afraid to touch her or the site of the surgery after it has healed. In the future you may need to massage (or touch) the area to promote a sense of normalcy. If you don't hesitate to touch the scar tissue and treat the area as you would any other portion of her body, it will help her accept the situation. You also may need to massage the area because it is common for phantom sensations to occur at the site of an amputation. Sometimes your wife may experience an itching on a portion of her missing breast. The sensation is real, just as if the breast is still there, and it is a very real problem. These sensations occur because the nerves, even though severed in surgery, still carry messages to the nerve endings and these messages translate into sensations. Briskly rubbing the area as if the breast were there often brings relief.

Touching your wife and participating in her healing promote reassurance while demonstrating your deep feelings for her. Also, it shows her that physical love is still very much a part of your life. Remember the old cliché: actions speak louder than words.

Andy: Unlike Bob and Martha, Ann and I took a bit longer before "the great unveiling."

It happened early one morning, about six weeks after Ann's surgery—as I helped her get dressed. In those days, Ann would towel off after her shower and then come out of the bathroom holding the big towel in front of her, as well as wearing a bathrobe. I would help her don certain items of clothing because the surgery had temporarily hampered her arm movement. She would hold on to the towel to prevent me from seeing her chest.

The entire process took loads of time and we mostly run late in the mornings anyway. This particular morning, Ann's arm got stuck while going through the routine. The bathrobe was half-on, half-off, and this big towel was preventing me from freeing her arm. I got a bit frustrated and yanked the towel out of the way, exposing Ann's chest.

This stunned her and she started hollering her head off for me not to look at her. At first I held her close to me, then I held her back so I could see the scars. I took a good look. Then I told her everything was okay.

"So, I saw your scars. I'm still here. I'm not taking gym shoes and heading for a divorce lawyer!" I exclaimed. I then told her I was going to take another look, prior to pushing her back gently but firmly, and took another good look as she continued to protest, but not as much as the first time. By now her anger had turned to tears of anguish.

My heart went out to Ann, not because of her scars, but because of her despair. I pulled her close again and hugged the daylights out of her.

The scars were not nearly so bad as I thought they'd be, and I told Ann so. In fact, they were not one hundredth as bad as my appendix scar, which Ann claims smiles at her from time to time, depending on how much I weigh.

Slowly her tears turned to ones of relief, joy, and thanksgiving. I'm sure Ann felt loved and so did I. There was also an added attraction. I found I could get much closer to Ann's heart than ever before and I got to listen to that big heart of hers beat and beat.

I'm also happy to report that since Ann's surgery, the so-called scars have almost disappeared. There is no indenture, and other than making Ann look like a very young girl, the scars are hardly noticeable. I think she even puts a bit of makeup on whatever scars remain. There are times, though, when Ann looks at herself and gets a bit down about what used to be there. But it's nothing a hug can't cure.

FOUR WAYS TO HELP HER AFTER SURGERY

We have discovered four general areas in which you can help your wife during these critical emotional times. A couple of the suggestions will appear to be patently obvious. And that's our challenge to you: Study the obvious and then implement it. We don't know your wife or her emotional needs, but we do know that generally life's greatest joys fall into the simplest categories. We hope that these four areas will make your love and devotion obvious to your wife while you search out and discover new ways to support her.

1. Be at the hospital as much as possible.

If you have young children, make arrangements for someone to take care of them. Keep your household in order so that you can devote time to your wife. You may have to work a job, go to the hospital to visit your wife, and then come home and clean up the house and see to it that the kids have clean clothes for school. But keep your priorities in the right order. Any household work can be achieved after—not during—hospital visiting hours. Any time they will let you in that hospital, you be there. No one knows your wife better than you, so be sensitive to her needs. And you may have to make some personal sacrifices to accommodate her wishes.

Andy: I wanted to be with Ann every second she was in the hospital but I put her wishes above mine that first night after surgery. Ann asked me to take her parents home and stay with

them. Since both her mother and father are elderly and have problems with their hearts, Ann wanted me to keep them calm and look after them in case of an emergency.

I was all set to tell Ann that this was one promise I just couldn't keep, as wild horses could not drag me from her bedside; then I reconsidered. It didn't take wild horses. It was just a simple request, but more than that; it was what Ann needed.

"This is very important to me. If you're not looking after Mom and Dad, then I'll be worried about them and you don't want me to have any additional worries," Ann had said to me on the way to the hospital. "Jean will take care of me at the hospital. But you're the only one I can completely trust to care for my parents."

Now, wild horses couldn't keep me from taking care of them. Sure, her words made me feel very important, but more importantly, I wanted to be as helpful as possible at a time I was needed, so I respected Ann's wishes. It became my daily responsibility to take her parents to the hospital and in the evening, I took them home and made sure they had a meal and were okay.

I am very proud of Ann for her caring and concern for others at a time when most of us would be thinking (and rightly so) only of ourselves. That's why, when people tell me how lovely Ann is, I always say: "You're right. But her beauty starts inside in that big heart of hers and works its way to the outside."

2. If your job or vacation time permits—and your wife doesn't have another job in mind for you—then stay with her.

Be her nurse. Dress her wounds, cajole her into eating, be helpful. Walk her around the floor or take her on leisurely strolls through the hospital grounds, stopping often for rest. Read a book out loud, play games, watch television; the list is endless. Spoil her with your loving attention and cater to her needs.

Now is not the time for false modesty. If there is anything she needs done physically, then do it. If you've never helped another use a bedpan or cleaned up a mess, now is the time to learn. Too often men have the tendency to consider certain things "woman's work." That phrase should no longer exist for you (if it ever did). Put yourself second and constantly think of what will make your wife more comfortable or content.

Besides helping her, you will be surprised to discover what this will do for *you!* Obviously it's an excellent way to demonstrate your love; but more than that, it has its own reward in that you are doing something for her. You have become a part of the recovery team. You no longer have to stand aside and let the doctors and the nurses care for her, as you look on feeling like an outsider. Participating in her care will help ease your stress and bolster your confidence because you are in the thick of the fight and can see daily improvement. Even the simplest activities take on special meaning, and if you can't think of anything to do for her, then simply sit in the room and hold her hand.

Bob: When Martha was fourteen, she was a sock-hop, bebop teen who disdained country music.

One day a friend offered Martha a double date with this real cute young man who was appearing on the Big D Jamboree, a country/western show in Dallas.

Leery, Martha asked the guy's name.

"Elvis," was her reply. "Elvis Presley."

"Elvis," Martha exclaimed, her teen dignity equally offended by that nerdy-sounding name and the country music he sang. "Who would ever, ever date a guy named Elvis?"

It was only a matter of months before "Blue Suede Shoes" made Elvis a national institution.

Like millions of other women, she followed his career, with an interest made unique by a teenage decision.

About the time of Martha's hospitalization, Elvis and Me was published. It was my task to read aloud to help while away those long hospital hours and it fell to me—a non-Elvis fan—to learn more about him than I ever cared to know.

Not only did I read the book to her, but we spent many hours discussing Elvis's career, his charisma, and decisions made by the many interesting people who populate the pages of the book.

One time I was reading away, my voice booming out dialogue, when a nurse came to the door, laughed, and shook her head.

"Will you two keep it down in here. This is a hospital. Some people are sick," she half-teased, half-fussed at us.

It became a fun time for both of us—and I even became a fan, of sorts—as we exchanged ideas, argued pros and cons on the King's career, and attempted to understand how wealth and fame seemed to ruin a performer who by all descriptions was just a simple man at heart when he first began to perform.

One thing Martha did say that touched my heart: "I never had a father read aloud to me. When you read, it makes me feel just like a little girl, safe and secure."

Ann turned an outpouring of love into a daily journey of joy. Gifts poured into the hospital room and flowers spilled into the hallway because of her celebrity status. Thousands of letters arrived daily at the hospital and at their home. In typical fashion, Ann shared with everyone.

Andy: Ann used to do her road work walking the halls and giving away lots of her flowers to other patients who did not have visitors very often. One time she worked up enough courage to walk into the late John Huston's suite when he was hospitalized for pulmonary emphysema, and gave him flowers. The famed director of such classics as *The Maltese Falcon* and *Treasure of the Sierra Madre* did not recognize her but enjoyed the flowers just the same. Ann got a giggle out of giving him the flowers because she was in such awe of the man and his work.

I found myself sneaking gourmet caviar in for Ann. The main thing is do whatever your wife needs done.

One of the benefits of spending time together and standing together in a common fight is that you and your wife should be drawn closer together; you could even fall in love again. We found this to be true in our own lives. Both of us have experienced a deeper love for our wives than we ever thought possible.

And along with this came a new appreciation. Character traits or abilities that you only suspected were there—in both of you—may begin to surface.

Andy: I got to see sides of my wife that I had always suspected were there, but had never witnessed until she was in this life-and-death situation.

Most of us never get the chance to be as great as we can be and to show ourselves and others all that we are capable of accomplishing.

It's like I used to tell many of the rookie police officers working under me when I was a sergeant on the Chicago police force: "Don't try to be a hero. When a situation calls for you to act, we will see whether or not you are a hero."

Ann and Martha, our wives, have had occasion to show what they are made of. They have risen to that occasion, and then some. Along with their actions comes a deepening respect from us and from their fellow humans. Any husband seeing this stuff in his lady knows that it makes for a very proud "I'm-glad-she's-married-to-me" feeling.

3. Be sensitive to your wife's emotional needs.

Your loving, special attention helps her cope. Besides being proud, don't forget to tell your wife how much you love her. Remember those days when you were courting? Remember how earnestly you tried to tell her the depth of your love? Now is the time to tell her—and show her—again. If you've gotten out of the habit, then make an extra effort. Wax poetic;

send her cards, candy, flowers, etc. She'll be glad you did and we know you'll be glad you did. Court her.

And you need to make her feel that she comes first in everything.

Andy: One day Ann was scheduled for her "lunchtime chemotherapy buffet" at the doctor's office and she was just too tired to take another dose of that stuff. As I slowly drove to the session, I could see her dread. I knew that she was thinking about another bad night. I also knew that what she needed was a "stay" of execution.

So, when we got to the doctor's office, there was a slight delay because all the chemo rooms were full. I used this "excuse" to start a petty beef with the doctor's staff.

"You know we're on a tight schedule. We're here and if you can't handle her needs, I'll just take her elsewhere," I said. In short I started a fight and fled the office with my Ann in tow. A smile begin to spread across her face as we ran to the car and drove to a restaurant.

Ann and I had a *real* lunch and we knew there would be no bad chemo night ahead for her. I felt like my wife's hero as she clung to my arm, both of us seated on the same side of the booth while we ate some of our favorite things. We were in love and very happy.

Now, I don't advise others to do this; appointments should be kept. And, yes, I rescheduled Ann for chemotherapy the very next day. But she did have a pleasant "stay."

4. Religious faith should not be overlooked.

It can be a powerful force. All four of us believe our faith helped us through our crisis.

We suggest that you take a look at your own faith to see if it can be a source of strength during *your* crisis. This can be a time of spiritual growth as you both find yourselves rethinking your priorities. Don't be afraid to turn to religion in your time of need.

Andy: I was not a big guy on faith. Although I was raised a Roman Catholic and married in a church, I never really got into the habit of attending, much less praying on a regular basis.

But when I was scared to the core, the first thing I did was kneel at the altar and make a deal with the Lord. If He would please spare Ann's life, I would straighten up. I knew that if she lived, her life would be an example.

When I told Bob about it, he chuckled with understanding and then told me about that old World War II axiom: "There are no atheists in foxholes."

Was he ever right.

The power of prayer should not be underestimated. If you attend religious services together, now is an excellent time to pray together. If you do not attend church, but your wife does, now is a wonderful opportunity for you to learn how to pray with her. She'll welcome the support and the strength. If you can't pray, then ask a minister or rabbi or the hospital chaplain to visit and lead you in prayer. It might also be time for you to go with her to a service.

If you read aloud to her, you might try a few of the comforting psalms found in the Bible. The well-known Twenty-third Psalm seems to be everyone's favorite. It certainly touches on both your needs at this time.

Bob: Ironically, I found myself in a position to practice what I preach, since as a guest minister in the Church of Christ, I have often extolled the virtues of deep faith and trust in God. I prayed—"beg" might be a better word—for many long hours either by myself or with Martha.

And sometimes the only satisfying solace I could find was Sunday and Wednesday when I sat in a pew among fellow believers, holding Martha's hand.

We believe we understand the words of the great prophet Jeremiah when he wrote (Jer. 10:23): "O Lord, I know that the way of man is not in himself; it is not in man that walketh to direct his steps."

BE READY TO MAKE CHANGES

Be prepared for anything. Your wife is probably in the most vulnerable emotional state of her life. If she has been an aggressive, take-charge "superwoman" in the past, you might be surprised to find that she now has difficulty making even the smallest decision, expecting instead for you to make most of the decisions while she hides behind your protective shield. On the other hand, a wife who has relied on her husband for everything may now decide to assert herself and may demand to make all of the decisions, fearing that a wrong one could cost her her life.

It has been our experience that the former change generally occurs. And it makes sense. Your wife is in the midst of a desperate struggle to survive. Information is piling up, many important decisions need to be made, and there is the constant worry about making a wrong choice. She knows her own emotional state and that knowledge in itself can breed anxiety. So, she turns to you for everything. If your wife can't trust you to help her make the right choices, then whom can she trust? Therefore, it is important that you work through the whole process with her.

Andy: It was confusing for me at first, because Ann went in the other direction. To a certain extent, she had always looked to me for everything, and I *loved* it. It made me feel important to her.

But then something happened. After all these years, Ann began making more decisions about her life and her career. I thought she had lost confidence in me. I felt hurt because as her personal manager, I had dedicated my life to her life. No one had ever questioned my ability, my trust, and especially my loyalty. Most criticism had centered on my being overly dedicated to her or my being overly protective. So, when Ann became this "new," assertive person, it baffled me.

All at once, she became extraordinarily opinionated on all aspects of her life. Her opinions on career moves shocked me the most. My gentle Annie wanted me to tell off this agent or

that person (if they had it coming). She wanted to let them know that she was not about to take any role just because it was offered. If it was not fun and exciting, she didn't want to do it. She is one dynamic businesswoman who has changed her stance, but not her respectful approach, in business dealings.

After my initial apprehension wore off, I came to realize that Ann's reasons for this change had nothing to do with my ability to handle her business affairs. Her outlook on life had changed and this "new," more confident Ann makes me even prouder than I was of the "old" Ann. And when I hear her give "what for" to some jerk in a business deal, or tell her agent exactly what she expects, there is no pussy-footing around. But I must say that she always has tact and a personal respect for the other person, two things I was short of from time to time.

What brought about this change? I don't know for sure, but in my talks with Ann, she says that after her battle with breast cancer, she felt the need to take firm control over her health and she also felt the need to have more control over her life and her career. And that meant helping me run our "mom and pop" business.

A side benefit to this is that Ann now trusts me more than ever. Our partnership is really much more equal than it was before. Now we are full-fledged partners in everything. Talk about happy!

Be prepared for just about any change in your wife's behavior. She may lash out at you in frustration. Because you love her—and because you have supported her so far—you are the safest person for her to attack verbally. Sometimes her angry outbursts are nothing more than venting her frustrations at her difficult situation.

Your wife might develop an interest in something that, until this moment, has been completely foreign to the "old" her. Although you may think you know everything there is to know about your wife, you may find her revealing emotions and thoughts that she never did before. And you may find yourself on the receiving end of some extraordinary conversations.

Bob: *"I don't want you to spend the money we've worked for and saved on another woman." Martha dropped this little bombshell on me as we were driving to the bank a few days before her first mastectomy. Her mother had died the year before, leaving her a modest inheritance, which I insisted be kept in her name. Now, facing the unknown, she wanted to add my name. I didn't want to do it, but agreed in an effort to keep her stress level as low as possible. We were on the way to the bank when this thought popped out.*

It didn't come as a surprise. Martha has been the financial mainstay of our family. I know of very few purchases she ever made at full price. Shopping with coupons is her way of life. Years ago, she practiced the kind of thrift that would later be extolled in a number of popular "how-to" books on family finances. Since I was a natural spendthrift, we often clashed over money during our lean, early years.

We had agreed that Martha would be a housewife, devoting her time to rearing our children and making a happy home. Meanwhile, we would live on whatever I could earn. We didn't exactly do that. Martha developed a number of money-making talents. She did baby-sitting, filling our home with children most days. Sometimes she took photos for newspapers, and other times she worked as a stringer, writing stories for newspapers in Houston and Waco.

"I've seen what happens to men after their wives die and they go crazy over younger women," she continued.

That didn't surprise me either. We'd had occasion to observe friends and acquaintances in similar circumstances.

"I want my children to get their inheritance from me. I've worked hard to put it together," she sighed.

I really didn't know what to do. I didn't like this kind of talk, but I understood what she was saying. If anything happened to me, she would automatically get everything we owned. But me? I was employed and didn't need any special financial care. Then it dawned on me.

I reached over and took her hand.

"Honey, you get hold of a CPA and have him put a dollar

value on everything we have," I said, listing rent property, savings, insurance, household furnishings, jewelry, cameras, etc. "After you get that, divide that figure in two. If we don't have that amount, we'll borrow it and put it in a savings account in your name only.

"You can make a will and if anything happens to you, then it will automatically go to the kids."

She looked at me and didn't say anything for a few seconds as she considered the offer.

"If you're willing to do that, then I don't want to," she replied.

She's never mentioned it again; but she knows the offer still stands.

So be prepared—you may hear some rather amazing things.

START PLANNING FOR THE FUTURE

Persuade her to make plans for the future. Everyone should have something to look forward to. This can be a real challenge. For years, both of you may have talked about retiring together, building a dream home, or taking a trip across the United States or to some exotic foreign land. Now, all of a sudden, your future has a lid on it. Instead of death being something that will happen in the distant future, it's *now* a real threat. Don't let this overburden your wife. Always speak in hopeful terms.

Start planning something. Is a child nearing graduation from high school or college? Is a grandchild about to be born? Is a job promotion or an anniversary near? How about a trip? You know your wife, so choose the place that will appeal to her.

Andy: Getting my wife to plan for the future is a very easy task. You see, Ann is an eternal optimist. She would probably

be planning a shopping trip if she were a convicted felon strapped into the electric chair!

Ann is the world's best list-maker. She has lists about lists. Her little lists are made on planes going to and from gigs, in car rides, and always around a magazine (she buys them all). And she has plenty of "honey-do" for me. There's always a room to be remodeled, a piece of furniture to be refinished, or a vacation to plan. We used to let work interfere with these things, but no more. We go on vacations and to hell with work!

Some of our research indicates that cancer survivors tend to be strong-willed people with unfinished business. If your wife doesn't have any plans or unfinished business, then it won't hurt for you to make some plans for her or to invent some unfinished business. She needs a sense of purpose in her life now more than ever.

Bob: Fortunately Martha and I had several upcoming events to plan for. Our daughter, Lilánd, was only a few months from graduating from high school when Martha's cancer was diagnosed. Despite her severe reaction to the chemotherapy treatments, Martha coordinated a graduation party for more than sixty guests, including family from out of town. Martha helped Lilánd shop for a prom dress, then bought herself a dress for the graduation. During long periods of rest at home in bed, due to exhaustion brought on by the chemotherapy, Martha organized her family into a cohesive party machine for the upcoming festivities.

A year later, we joined my sister, Nancy, in throwing a party for my parents' fiftieth wedding anniversary. Martha and I decided to observe our twenty-fifth wedding anniversary quietly.

In one of those ironies of life, on the day we celebrated our anniversary Martha was told that a second biopsy would be required in her remaining breast. It was also on that day that Martha decided to go ahead and have the second mastectomy even if no cancer was discovered, rather than spend years worrying about having a biopsy every time something suspicious showed on the X rays. It was a day of extreme emotion as we spent the evening at home, holding hands and reviewing the past years.

"I didn't think I'd be here for this," she said of our twenty-fifth anniversary. It had been almost two years to the date that we'd begun the battle.

Martha's next gala event was a big bash in honor of our son, Bobby, who was receiving his D.D.S. degree from the University of Texas Health Science Center, after seven years of study.

As time passes, the need for goals lessens. But I still occasionally throw one out, just to be safe.

FIGHTING DEPRESSION

Special activities and plans will help fight your biggest emotional foe: depression. Some women feel ashamed because they suffer symptoms of depression. They shouldn't. It is, perhaps, the most common reaction. Several cancer victims have told us that the best money they spent was on a psychiatrist, who helped them sort out their feelings. Don't forget that you, too, may want to seek professional help from a psychiatrist or psychologist—for either you or your wife; or your children.

No matter how upbeat, how perky or how optimistic the patient, there will still be times of depression. If it progresses too far, then you will need some outside help.

"If you think about it, in broad strokes, just about anyone going through this type of crisis could use some help," one psychiatrist told us.

So, if you decide you need help, search out a psychologist or psychiatrist with the same diligence you used to obtain that second opinion for your wife. We suggest four sources that should prove helpful, even if you live in a small town.

1. Locate the nearest medical school and see if it has a department of psychiatry. It would be best if you could talk to the

head of the department, remembering to keep your visit brief. He or she can recommend several experts, perhaps some that he has even helped train or someone on his staff. One psychiatrist told us to be sure and get the names of several doctors because one may be too busy and you may not feel comfortable with another; this keeps your options open. Hint: Secretaries can be an invaluable help, no matter whom you are attempting to reach. When you first contact the department, ask the secretary if you can explain what your needs are. The secretary can then summarize everything for the head of the department, and thus speed up the search process.

2. Discuss your needs with a trusted medical expert such as the surgeon, oncologist, or family doctor who is treating your wife.

3. Often a minister acts as a counselor and also knows members of the medical community who offer psychiatric help. The minister may have recommendations for you.

4. Check with the local or county association of mental health experts. The nearest medical school could put you in touch with the local mental health organization. The local branch of the American Medical Association would know of such an organization, too, as would the American Psychiatric Association. If these fail, pick up the telephone, call any of the psychologists or psychiatrists in the Yellow Pages, and ask them the name and telephone number of the local organization.

And finally, insist that the expert you choose be board-certified.

How can you tell if you or your wife is depressed enough to warrant professional help? It takes years of study for a person to become a licensed psychiatrist or psychologist, so we certainly aren't experts. But we can give you a broad outline that we hope will be a guide.

Generally speaking, there are people who are in a state of being depressed and people who are in depression. The big difference is that *being depressed* happens for a brief period of time and people snap back; *depression* is a cluster of symptoms that are sustained for a minimum of two weeks and that cause dysfunction.

Being depressed is a mood change best described as "being down," in the blahs, sad, blue, or indifferent, listless; it can last for a few minutes, a few hours, or maybe a day or two before a person charges headlong back into life.

Depression, on the other hand, is a set of symptoms—including mood changes—that can sometimes be triggered by physical reactions to medical treatment. Aside from prolonged mental anguish, there is the "global syndrome," causing either too much or too little sleep, too much or too little appetite, agitation or lethargy, fatigue, a loss of sex drive, memory lapses, nervousness, tension, and such severe withdrawal that one no longer wants to socialize or see visitors. Psychiatrists have told us that biochemical changes, from both the cancer and the treatments, can help cause depression.

A woman facing breast cancer may feel negative, helpless, hopeless, filled with a sense of doom. These feelings can be so profound that a person wishes for the relief of death, as Martha did on the day of biopsy.

She may express an excessive sense of guilt, reaching back into her past to dredge up old, long-forgotten misdeeds and feeling guilty for them.

Sometimes there is a loss of self-esteem. She may see herself as a sort of modern-day leper; a blight has hit her, she is doomed and unworthy to be part of the human race.

The key question is, Is your wife being depressed or in depression? In layman's terms you can say that depression equals pessimism plus sadness. Is this happening to your wife? Experts tell us that along with mood changes, four major symptoms have to be present nearly every day for a period of at least two weeks for a person to be clinically considered in depression. Major symptoms include poor appetite or significant weight loss or significant weight gain; insomnia or hypersomnia; psychomotor agitation (pacing, restlessness, hand wringing, etc.) or retardation (slowed movements); loss of interest or pleasure in usual activities or decrease in sex drive; loss of energy or fatigue; feelings of worthlessness, self-reproach or excessive or inappropriate guilt; diminished ability to think or concentrate; indecisiveness; excessively pessimistic outlook, and recurrent thoughts of death.

One psychiatrist pointed out that due to the nature of the illness, most cancer patients are depressed but not *in* depression, so don't try to diagnose your wife. Just check the list and if she has enough of these symptoms to indicate she may need help, then get her to the proper expert. And while you're at it, check yourself, too.

Bob: Once the chemotherapy treatment got under way, depression became one of Martha's biggest problems. It came at her from two different directions. Naturally, there was the emotional ordeal of dealing with a life-threatening disease; just as insidious was the physical ordeal, which hampered her ability to fight the emotional battle.

Another problem was the very nature of the disease. Think of whatever is your worst fear. (Mine would be to lose my eyesight.) Martha's worst fear had always been cancer. And now, not only did she have to face it, but also she had to learn to live with it. It was an enormous emotional burden.

Couple this with chemotherapy and/or radiation treatments, which lower a person's natural defenses, and you have someone who is in a weakened, vulnerable condition. Sometimes Martha's depression stemmed from being physically unable to get out of bed or handle her routine chores. She was struggling to maintain a positive mental attitude but her weakened physical condition made it more difficult for her.

Then one day we developed a twenty-five-year plan. Don't ask me why twenty-five years, it just seemed like a good number. I was desperate to help her and suggested this.

"Look, you can be depressed and cry and be miserable and wake up twenty-five years from now and have had a lousy life; wasted," I told her. "Or, you can live each day, happy to be with your family, and wake up twenty-five years from now

and have had a wonderful life. And, should anything happen between now and twenty-five years, at least those will have been happy years for us."

So we decided to live each day to its fullest—to enjoy life and to stop and smell the roses. We've always enjoyed each other's company, but now our time together seems even more special. We're grateful for what we have and in twenty-five years we will be more grateful still.

At the same time we decided to visit a psychiatrist in an effort to get a handle on the situation. I didn't know about the depression checklist at the time, but there were enough symptoms that my instincts told me we needed help. Through a skillful combination of medication and counseling, a psychiatrist helped Martha turn the tables on depression. It was not an overnight victory and it took time and work, but soon Martha was welcoming visitors instead of turning them away; awaking each morning to accept the challenge of each day; and taking nourishment.

We do have a minor disagreement on this. She doesn't believe the sessions helped her all that much; I saw such an immediate improvement in her fighting spirit that I believe they did. But when she wanted to stop after three or four sessions, I agreed because I didn't believe it fair to push her.

I don't believe it matters if we agree or not over the treatment. What does matter is that she made it through these troubled times.

By all means be sure to check your insurance policy. Many companies pay a set, yearly amount or will cover half or more of treatment costs. And if your insurance won't help pay, other financial help may be available. Contact your local United Way for a list of members or the American Cancer Society for a list of agencies that can provide financial help or services.

Months, even years later, depression will continue to rear its head, so be prepared to deal with it over the long haul. It won't hurt to spend a little time in thought, preparing yourself.

What do you say if you discover your wife secretly crying in the bathroom? What challenge can you give her that will fill her thoughts with resolve and anticipation? What words will swiftly reassure her of your love and your future together?

Other times your wife will have the situation under control only to be staggered by tragedy, such as the unexpected death of a friend or, even worse, the death of a friend to cancer. When this happens, it may trigger feelings of depression long after you thought they were gone.

Andy: Whenever I see a little tear creeping down Ann's cheek (I have to tell you these times are so rare now it's hard to remember when it last happened), I encourage her to talk to me.

When the tears appear, it is usually after a shower. If I don't hear the usual noises, I turn down the TV and listen. If a few minutes go by, I holler, "Are you okay, babe?" And, if I don't get a quick response, I go into the bathroom and hug Ann, and she has a little cry. I only need to hold Ann and tell her I love her and all is okay. Then I point out that God gave her life so we could be together as a family, with her mom and dad and brother.

Many times I've tried to explain my feelings to Ann, but the best chance came one afternoon while we were filming an appearance on "Hour Magazine," a television talk show. We had been discussing Ann's case and a woman's feelings about the loss of her breasts, when Gary Collins, the show's host, turned to me and asked:

"How about you, Andy. How is all this affecting you?"

I wanted to answer that question and somehow put Ann's mind at ease while being helpful to the thousands of men and women facing a similar problem. I was holding Ann's hand at the time and I lifted it into the air.

"If my wife had to lose some part of her anatomy, I would prefer it be those breasts with cancer than this hand I'm holding," I said, turning to look into Ann's eyes. I could tell Ann felt the truth of what I had said. She squeezed my hand and tears appeared in her eyes. After the show she confessed: "You stole my heart all over again when you said that today."

BATTLING STRESS

We don't believe that we can put too much stress on stress. Our experiences and discussions with fellow fighters indicate that stress will now play a predominate role in your life. Common sense tells you that fighting any major illness is stressful; but it seems to us that fighting breast cancer is especially stressful because of the disfigurement and life-and-death struggle it entails. The physical illness alone places tremendous stress on the mind and body. There's also the strain of awaiting test results, and postoperative and treatment recuperation. Added to these is "waiting for the other shoe to drop"—the fear of cancer recurring—that is a part of living with this disease.

For years, just the mention of breast cancer struck terror into the hearts of healthy women. Thankfully, mastectomies are no longer mentioned only in hushed tones or whispered about at sewing circles or over the backyard fence. In this country, mastectomies are a reality of life and a woman who has had a mastectomy can be just as sensual, vibrant, and alive as other women. Because of a newfound perspective, she may actually enjoy life more than she ever has once she has learned to manage stress.

Managing stress could mean a change of values—for both of you. It's inconceivable that you two could go through this ordeal unchanged. Life will be constantly changing now; new values will surface and possibly new priorities.

Andy: Ann and I decided to "stop and smell the roses." It was an easy decision to make, because all we really had to do was drop something that had been with us all of our ten years of marriage: trying to make it to the top.

It consumed our lives. We lived each day for it. We made our friends in the business. Success was all we thought of and

worked so hard for, and it always seemed to be just a movie or a television series away.

Ann had some wonderful successes. Her work in *Mae West* was nominated for an Emmy and a Golden Globe. She received a second Emmy nomination for the miniseries *Ellis Island* and a third Emmy nomination for her role in *The Ann Jillian Story.* But each year someone else won the big award and it was pick up and start all over again.

It was a tough way to live and we now believe that the stress Ann was under all the time "trying to make it" was or could have been a factor in getting breast cancer. Who knows?

Right after Ann's surgery, we got smart and changed our lives.

"I'm Ann Jillian's director of entertainment," I told her agent one morning. I explained that from now on we would plan vacations (we had never done this before) and I would see to it that she no longer would do any work that she didn't want to do. The first thing I wanted her to do was drop her role in the series "It's a Living." For many reasons, it had become stressful and we now had new priorities in our lives. We wanted to experience life—live and enjoy each other—as much as we could after her surgery. There was no longer the all-consuming need to make it big.

What good would all the money and fame have done us if Ann had died from breast cancer? These things could never be a substitute for life.

We decided to reclaim our priorities by cutting out certain things that were no longer important to us. First to go was that series and all its stress. Ann no longer had to go into that big cave of a studio at sun-up and return home well after dark. She no longer had to miss her backyard and all her flowers.

We cut back on most of the publicity stuff such as interviews and photo sessions in which we tried to be in the news by keeping a high profile. We took a lower profile. Ann still does publicity for each individual project, but after that it's right back to her flowers.

We try not to book one project right after the other. We try to make room in between for very important rest and relaxation. We strive to keep stress at a minimum. We watch her diet, make sure she gets plenty of exercise and that she is checked every three months, although her doctor says once a year is enough. The frequent checkups are my idea and it gives both of us peace of mind. We learned our lesson about early detection. Catch it soon enough and you live.

We want life and we want a good quality of life. We also now work only with nice people. If they are difficult, we don't go near them. No sum of money is worth being in a situation where one is stressed and unhappy. Health is too important to us now.

If possible, cut out the bad things in your life. You as a husband might have to quit that second job so you can spend a little more time with your wife. If you two are happy, then to hell with the new car. Fix the old one! Our new values say that a simple life is the best.

All the experts suggest that your life be reordered to eliminate as much stress as possible. There is a popular theory concerning stress that is gaining attention in medical and psychological circles. And although the jury is still out—and doubtlessly will be for a number of years—it is worthy of consideration.

The theory concerns the effects of stress and depression on the human body. Some experts believe that stress may promote the development of cancer by hampering the immune system's functioning. Scientists do agree that stress can hamper the immune system. Some breast cancer patients had either suffered stress or experienced one or more traumatic events between one to two years before the appearance of breast cancer. Examples of traumatic experiences cited are the death of an authority figure (such as a mother or father), death of a spouse or child, a child leaving home, loss of a job (either husband or wife), a life-threatening accident, or a divorce. The theory holds that such emotional upheavals can lead to a deep depression, which in turn can lead to suppression of the immune system, which daily kills malfunctioning cells that turn into cancer.

The theory further states that each person handles stress in his or her own unique way; therefore, some people are at higher risk than others. We have to be careful here because we are *not* saying that everyone is going to get cancer because of a traumatic experience. Obviously each person handles adversity in a different manner.

But you have to be careful and not overreact. One woman determined after mastectomy that it was her husband who caused her cancer because living with him was too stressful. To his amazement, she divorced him.

Bob: This has become almost a personal crusade for me. I don't know if the theory is true or not—and most medical experts are skeptical—but I know that whenever I ask a women to consider the eighteen to twenty-four months before diagnosis, with very few exceptions they all recall traumatic times. (I'm aware that life is a continuing process, often layered with trying times, and that most people can cite emotional upheavals within the last twelve to eighteen months of their lives. I realize that, but I still believe there is something here.)

Martha lost her mother about eighteen months before her diagnosis. At the same time, I went through a job-threatening incident, and I was involved in an accident with a roto-tiller in which only Martha's quick action saved my leg from being mangled. It was a rough period for her.

The point is—whether the theory is true or not—we know that no good can come from stress. Now that Martha has successfully negotiated cancer treatment, I do everything I can to keep stress at a minimum, even if it means standing between her and family obligations. My cousin who was dying of cancer asked me to conduct her funeral service. I was honored to be asked, and Martha was ready to do whatever was necessary. But I asked Martha not to attend the services because I felt it would be depressing and she acquiesced to my request. My family understood and agreed with my actions.

You need to know when to shield your wife from stressful situations. But sometimes you have to take your cue from her to make sure you aren't being too overprotective.

Andy: From time to time fans of Ann's come up to her or mail her photos that display her former cleavage.

At first I used to try to keep those photos from Ann. I felt it would remind her of her breasts and put her into a slight melancholic state. And I was right. It did. Ann told me so. But she kept right on signing those photos and thanked her fans for asking for her autograph.

One day we got to talking about this business and she related to me that at first she did get a bit down in the dumps.

"I realized that it was part of my business, and it was not about to go away," she said. "I was slightly suspicious when fans sent me pictures that revealed my cleavage.

"I must admit I was hoping that they wanted me to sign because they liked my work and it was the only picture they had of me—not because they wanted a 'souvenir' of my former breast tops."

After a while, Ann got used to it.

"Whenever I see the tops of my breasts now, it's like visiting a couple of good friends; family, actually," Ann laughed.

To some degree, stress is subjective. Jumping out of an airplane may be the ultimate in fun and relaxation for a sky diver, but it would be stressful for most of us. So, take a few minutes to consider what contributes to stress in your life. The obvious causes are easy to tag: fears, feeling hopeless or out of control, the unknown, etc. Now, search out the subtle stresses in your own situation, which may be beginning to build. You need to spot these and to try to defuse them. You will need to schedule moments of rest and relaxation for your wife. Help her reshape her perspective. Some people get so caught up in the urgency of the moment that they lose sight of the big picture.

You will need staying power for the long haul. Staying power is the ability to put yourself on "hold"—idling your motor when you feel like stripping the gears.

Andy: Ann really did not get depressed to the extent that she needed professional care. Sure there were moments when she would be showering and I'd hear a sniffle or two, but as she says, "I was so glad just to be alive that I found I did not get seriously depressed." There's a big difference between depression and being down in the dumps.

In fact, I used to keep a lot of women and well-meaning folks away from Ann because their comments about others only made Ann think twice about the way she was handling it all. I thought, "Hey, if she ain't down and she has a handle on it, let well enough alone."

Ann scared me. I thought she bounced back so fast because she was worried about her elderly parents and about me. But apparently not, at least not completely. It was her way of handling it.

She wasn't being just a "good soldier" when she returned to work on "Alice in Wonderland" in eleven days. She wanted to finish her work because it meant that "even though I was just told that I had in fact had cancer, my life was already going right on in spite of it." I almost think Ann felt that if she had stopped at any of these roadblocks, she would have been stopping her life and giving in to cancer.

Later we came to believe that it was her subconscious way of telling cancer to get lost; that there would be no lying down today without a good, old-fashioned fight.

It also kept her head in the right place and allowed her to feel useful and productive. Also, in Ann's business, had she ducked out of the "scene," rumors would have been rampant that she was all but dead.

Me? I got depressed. While Ann's experience with cancer had been positive, mine had been tragic. I went to a shrink for his advice on how to handle this thing both for me and for Ann. I wanted to help her all I could, but I had to keep myself straight, first. He helped me cope with the reality of my mom and sister dying of cancer and my fears that Ann might die, too.

Ann was looking into my eyes and instead of seeing life and spark, my eyes were saying, "So this is how we are to part!" This was the worst thing I could do. Ann didn't want sympathy, she wanted to see some fight in my eyes, the same as in hers.

I came around fast. The shrink told me that life should go on normally. He told me to see to it that Ann received proper medical care and that she followed through.

"Then you both have to get on with your life," he said. "Try to get off alone from time to time, reduce your work load, rest and relax more."

I knew what the doctor was saying was right. Even Jesus Christ would escape the stresses of the work-a-day world. He would leave the crowds and go into the mountains, or board a boat to escape the crowds demanding his attention. He would rest—refresh himself—and let others serve Him before returning to his work.

"Enjoy life more, not because you think Ann might die, but because there is life and life is meant to be lived," he continued.

We decided to take it a day at a time. The way I figure it, if cancer is going to kill anyone else in my family, it will have to do it while we are living it up and not while we are sitting around worrying about it.

To this day I can't talk about possible death from cancer. I just can't handle it. But this also gives me the strength to give others hope and not let them defeat themselves.

There is nothing "sissy" about seeing a psychiatrist for help. He helped me set myself straight so I could help the woman I love.

9

Exercise and Nutrition

EXERCISE

Be sure that your wife gets proper exercise and nutrition both during hospitalization for surgery, chemotherapy treatment, and as she recovers. A sensible program, followed faithfully every day, will help strengthen her body, speed recovery, and may help buoy her spirits. But don't expect results overnight. Common sense tells you to take it slow and not to do anything unless the doctor orders it or approves.

The very first exercise will be in the hospital when she takes those initial faltering steps down the hallway. Gradually increase the length of the walk as she gains strength and confidence. Praise her efforts; point out her improvement with each trip, encourage her to take these walks. Pause often to let her rest, look out the windows at the rest of the world, which is awaiting her return, and talk about pleasant things, maybe something you two will do once she is out of the hospital.

By now she should have been visited by the Reach to Recovery volunteer who will teach her a full range of exercises. These simple exercises are compiled by experts and developed specifically for women who have had mastectomies. Just as importantly, the exercises will ease her back into a normal life. So, if she hasn't had a visit from Reach to Recovery, then encourage her to tell the doctor that she wants one.

Now begins the second set of exercises, which are designed to return full use of the arm. With very few exceptions, she will regain functional use, including the ability to raise her arm above her head. Many women suffer from a real fear that they have been permanently disabled and after watching our wives overcome the physical trauma, we can understand this fear. So be patient and extremely encouraging, pointing out each increment of improvement. We suggest that you try to set up a schedule of exercises based on the Reach to Recovery regimen of finger wall-walking, ball tossing, and hand-pumping above your head; perhaps four five-to-ten minutes segments each day. The exercises may look easy, but for a woman who has just had surgery, they can be difficult to perform. Meanwhile, keep up the brief walks once you reach home, but extend them into the neighborhood.

Andy: Ann found the shower to be very helpful when doing her exercises. She would turn the heat up—careful not to get it too hot—and steam up the room. Then, standing in the shower, she would walk her fingers up the wall, stretching her muscles and exercising the area of surgery. The heat and the steam seemed to help soften and stretch the muscles, making the exercise a little easier than when the skin was dry.

I also tried to make some of the exercises more fun. If she walked through a room I was in, I pointed my finger at her like a pistol, and barked in my best James Cagney voice, "Okay, Whitey, up with them." She then had to raise her arms as high as possible and do her hand-pump exercise.

Bob: *Just don't make the same mistake I did. I misunderstood and instead of letting Martha exercise at a more leisurely pace, I urged her higher and higher each session, marking new levels of achievement on the bedroom door. I noticed that the finger-walking caused her a great deal of pain,*

but believed we were doing good by stretching the muscles;
until the day she threw up from pain that became so intense
her stomach rebelled.

    Confused and angry, I called the doctor.

    "No," he patiently explained. "Let her go at her own pace.
She'll pick it up as she goes along."

Today, both women exercise. Ann is on a strict regimen
designed to keep her body trim for her career and also designed
to keep her from having to go through another year of the
intense exercise required to get into shape for filming *The Ann
Jillian Story.* Martha goes to a local health spa where she
swims, spends time in the steam room, and joins in floor exercises. She has found swimming to be her favorite exercise and
the most helpful for strengthening her arms. As often as she can
get Bob out the door, they take long brisk walks through the
neighborhood. During rainy weather they go to the mall to
walk.

It's difficult, at best, to follow a strict exercise program, so
we suggest that either you exercise with your wife or that you
help her find an exercise buddy or an organized exercise class.
Don't forget that she will need proper exercise clothing so she
won't be self-conscious. Leotards (pick your or her favorite
color) and a sharp-looking but loose-fitting top would make a
dandy gift—one of those "just because I love you" surprises.

If a YWCA or other health club is not in your budget, then
maybe you can rent or purchase an exercise video tape. Some
city libraries have them available to check out and you can
sample a number before deciding which one she wants. (This
would make an excellent birthday or Mother's Day gift.) Your
wife might want to explore the possibility of starting her own
exercise group.

Both of our wives experienced weight gain—we understand that some chemo drugs actually add pounds—that
caused consternation and experimentation with a series of
diets and, in Ann's case, a determined exercise program.

Andy: There is a lady named Luretta McCray, who is a singer/dancer and choreographer who works in Ann's concert act. She is a "health nut" in the best sense because she has common sense.

She teamed up with us to get Ann in shape and they went through a three-month program that still has my head spinning. Five days a week, three hours each day, Luretta would come to Ann's rehearsal studio behind our house.

Stop! Before you read any further, please understand that Ann did not start this tough schedule until she had been checked by the doctor and told it was safe to proceed. If you decide to exercise, visit your doctor, too. That's a must. Don't overdo it and injure yourself. You must set a realistic goal and work up to it a little at a time. That's an order from the sergeant.

Now, back to the story. Luretta established a pattern. The first hour was devoted to slow and easy stretches that warmed up their muscles. The second hour they would get into some hot exercising movements for those special areas of the body that many women have problems with—the hips, thighs, legs, and bottom.

This is where Luretta made it special. Like most people, Ann doesn't like to exercise just to exercise; so, Luretta used her talents as a choreographer to "fit" the exercise to dance music (Ann's favorite songs) and they would work each exercise as if it were a movement to be incorporated into an overall dance routine. Each step or movement was designed to help a problem area. Ann loved it! The last ten minutes of the second hour were devoted to putting it all together into a continuous dance routine just as if they were going to present it on a television special. The routine grew each day as a new movement was added and by the end of the three months, they had themselves a full-blown, wonderfully choreographed exercise that could have been put into Ann's act with the audience none the wiser.

The third hour was devoted to cooling off by using the life-cycle exerciser. Ann started at twelve minutes and built up to forty. Then they would practice relaxation techniques, unwinding to soft, soothing music. The session ended with Ann heading for a nice, steamy shower and a fluffy terry cloth robe.

Renee Sousa, singer/dancer in Ann's concert act and a licensed masseuse, sometimes would give Ann a massage to end an evening workout session.

It is only fair to point out that Ann's weight, when she went from a size six to sixteen, did not just melt away immediately after starting her diet and exercise program. As soon as she stopped taking chemo she worked out for one entire month on the five-day schedule and at the end of that time had gained one pound! Ann could not lose a pound for an entire year. No one, not even the doctor, could explain it. It seemed to us that Ann's body had to rid itself completely of the chemo drugs before it would respond to the exercise program and return to a normal weight almost two years later. Finally, after days and weeks of exercise, something happened and the weight started to come off. At thirty-eight, Ann knows that it only gets harder to lose weight as we get older, so she is steadfast about maintaining her present shape. It took hard, concentrated work for Ann to lose the extra pounds and to keep them off; she still uses that specially choreographed exercise routine, but now only two or three days a week for weight maintenance.

Like everyone else, Ann tried fad diets and fad exercises; but there is only one way to lose weight, and that is to *earn it off* the old-fashioned way. A good pair of wrists that can push you away from the dinner table do as much good as pushups. Add a commonsense diet and shed bad habits like you want to shed pounds.

Again, a word of caution. Before your wife starts any type of exercise program, demand that your doctor approve the specific routine she will follow.

NUTRITION

Your recovery program will call for a two-stage nutritional program.

First, you will need to help ensure proper nutrition following surgery and chemotherapy or radiation when nausea, and sometimes depression, cause a loss of appetite.

Second, you may have to change your eating habits when she returns to the work-a-day world with its fast foods, greasy and fried foods, and improper nutrition. And you may have to cope with a phenomenon that is not uncommon with women who have received chemotherapy: rapid weight gain. We watched with joy and then amazement as our wives emerged from the debilitating effects of chemotherapy and began to put on weight rapidly. We don't know if this need was physical (that the body wanted nourishment after a lean period) or mental (that there was a subconscious desire to treat and be kind to a body that had just gone through hell). But it soon became a major concern.

But first, let's look at the problem of proper nutrition during recovery.

A well-nourished body is nature's way of helping fight disease, thereby increasing the effectiveness of therapy and speeding recovery from treatment. A balanced diet high in protein, with extra vitamins and minerals from fruits, vegetables, and whole grains, helps patients withstand the side effects of treatment, maintain strength by rebuilding normal tissue that has been affected by treatment, and shore up the battered immune system. Common sense tells you that an undernourished body is vulnerable. If your wife was like Ann and Martha, she was in peak health when the cancer was discovered; so you start with a healthy body that is usually debilitated by treatment, although a patient will occasionally experience weight gain throughout the ordeal.

Don't be afraid to try almost anything to get her interested in food. Something as simple as an elegantly appointed dining table with a few fresh flowers or the smell of freshly baked bread may awaken an interest. Dining out or sharing a meal with friends or having a backyard picnic often helps.

Be prepared for her tastes to change. Favorite foods will no longer be favored. Something straight out of left field—such as potato salad—might hit the spot. A number of chemotherapy patients have told us that they lost their taste for red meat; it was more than a year before Martha could eat steak, until then her favorite food.

Andy: Something that worked for Ann throughout chemotherapy was a breakfast bowl of fruit, which I prepared fresh every morning.

First I would peel and divide oranges and grapefruit into sections. Next I would clean and slice apples—green and red— and arrange the pieces in a colorful way. Next came cantaloupe, which I would scoop out with my trusty "melon baller." Then, I'd slice in a nice banana and, if I had one, a little fresh pineapple. There you have it. Yellow, red, green, pink, orange, and maybe some seedless grapes to add a royal purple.

Now it's colorful enough for my queen to eat.

Ann loved it. And many mornings it soothed her tummy after a hard night.

My "Parade of Fruit" is still one of her favorite dishes. You might try it—only adjust it to your wife's taste.

She will experience a lot of general eating problems during treatment. Some people just don't eat as much because food doesn't taste right or because they just aren't hungry. Sometimes she may have to force herself to eat a number of small meals.

The topic of trying to eat while nauseous deserves a book and, in fact, a number have been written, including several distributed by the American Cancer Society and the National Cancer Society. Just about everything—sight, smell, taste, bloating, soreness in the mouth and throat—comes into play, so you have to carefully consider everything in light of your wife's specific needs.

Bob: You guessed it. There was absolutely nothing that could stay in Martha's stomach, especially the week following chemotherapy. It was a difficult time for her and she started losing weight. But the weight loss was not so worrisome as the chronic fatigue, which struck immediately. It was almost impossible for her to get out of bed and then only for brief periods.

The oncologist helped ease our anxiety about proper nutrition by adding liquid vitamins to Martha's IV following her chemo treatments at the hospital. If she wasn't getting protein, at least she was getting proper vitamins and nutrition.

I read that extremely cold drinks, such as ice cream and frozen ices, often were palatable, so I stocked the freezer and those items seemed to help. Anything icy cold went down easier.

Another trick I used was to make Martha drink a nutriment concoction, the type found in pharmacies and grocery stores and used to supplement baby diets (sometimes athletes drink them for quick energy). They are chock full of calories and vitamins, but have a pungent smell. Martha hated both the taste and the smell, so I would get it icy cold, pour about a third of a can into a glass, take it to her, and demand that she down it, just like taking medicine. She would—sometimes holding her nose, that's no exaggeration—and we would spend the next half-hour keeping it down. I'd massage her feet and talk to her about our safe place and beautiful beaches. Once she settled down, I'd get the next third, etc., until a small can had been consumed. A few hours later, there would be a blush to her cheeks and you could almost see the strength flowing into her body. She could feel the difference, and she knew that it helped her. That's about the only reason she gamely made herself consume it.

A few hours later, I'd be back with another can. It didn't make any difference if it was strawberry, vanilla, or chocolate, she hated them all.

I knew Martha was starting to recover when we attended a family gathering. She hadn't eaten for weeks, but for some reason the potato salad appealed to her and she ate plate after plate. Me? I turned into a potato salad-making fool.

There's going to be a transition from the time she starts gaining strength after treatment until she regains her position in the household. It's going to be a period of decision making concerning your lifestyle and eating habits. Your wife, your family, and you have come this far. Do you stop? That's up to you. But if you listen to the American Cancer Society, you'll give some careful thought to change. Again, it's just common sense. Would you deliberately do something that would cause recurrence? Stupid question, isn't it? There are nutritional suggestions approved by the ACS that offer potential prevention of cancer. It seems a good idea to us to follow that plan as closely as possible.

The seven-step ACS plan is simple and, by following it, you may lessen the chances of cancer.

1. Avoid obesity. (As we've discussed, many women tend to put on weight following chemotherapy.)

2. Cut down on total fat intake. A diet high in fat may be a factor in the development of cancer.

3. Eat more high-fiber foods in the form of cereals, fresh fruits, and vegetables. High-fiber foods are a wholesome substitute for foods high in fat.

4. Include foods rich in vitamins A and C in your daily diet. That means dark green and deep yellow fresh vegetables and fruits such as carrots, spinach, yams, acorn and butternut squash, peaches, and apricots for vitamin A. Choose oranges, grapefruit, strawberries, and green and red peppers for vitamin C.

5. Include cruciferous vegetables. That means cabbage, broccoli, brussels sprouts, kohlrabi, and cauliflower should be included in the menu.

6. Eat moderately of salt-cured, smoked, and nitrite-cured foods.

7. Keep alcohol consumption moderate or, better yet, cut alcohol out of your diet all together.

Bob: Men, you're in for a treat; and, ladies, I hope you're reading this section, too, because I'm turning this over to Andy. I can cook a bit, but it's generally out of a can or a box. My kids tagged me king of the hamburger helpers and I do claim a certain expertise in that particular cuisine. But Andy is something special. To me, he's a bit of a gourmet while my tastes are more pedestrian. Dining with Andy is an experience. He tries a little bit of this and a little of that until the table groans with food and he's urging you to eat more.

About the only diet tip I have is to urge that your wife take only half portions of any particular food. Have her determine how much she wants, and then take only half the amount—and I stole that tip from Andy.

———

Andy: First, nutrition. In general, I went back to a commonsense type of overall diet. I mean Mama's type of food such as fresh fruits, greens, vegetables, chicken and fish, and even a good steak now and then. The only problem is that it's hard to get this type of food nowadays. Most everything seems to be refined or processed or doused with poisons or injected with "grow faster"-type chemicals. I found myself doing a lot of research in my area—you do the same—to find the source of the same foods that Mama cooked for us when we were growing up. I was able to locate sources for fresh eggs, fresh vegetables, and even fresher water to cook them in.

Become a "washing nut." I wash *everything* before I cook it. You really don't know what it's been through or who handled it or what possible contagious disease that handler may have had. Do you want to play the "catch a germ wheel"? I think not. And perhaps if I can talk you into considering the possibility of germs on food, maybe you can consider what causes cancer? We really don't know, so as long as we don't know, why not try to keep the things we put in our bodies as clean as possible. So, while we're waiting to find out beyond a shadow of a doubt, let's clean up our act.

Next, plan hunting sprees. I prowl the various supermarkets, fruit stands, and groves to find the best fruits and vegetables that are in season. I do most of the food shopping because it is difficult for Ann. If she goes to the supermarket, she winds up signing autographs and visiting with her good fans—not that she minds, but she takes too long to get the basket full! Besides, being the chief cook and bottle washer is something I can "do" for Ann and not feel so helpless in this cancer battle and her recovery. So, I have turned into an excellent shopper and can be as aggressive as anyone else in going for the juiciest orange.

Breast cancer is one type of cancer that seems to be affected by diet and nutrition. Countries where there is a high fat content in the diet tend to have a high rate of breast cancer. Argentina is a good example. It is a country with a high rate of beef consumption and a high cancer rate. Asian countries with a diet low in beef and other fatty foods have a corresponding lower rate of breast cancer; but, if Asians migrate and start eating a diet high in fat, they start getting breast cancer at an increased rate.

I'm not saying we should all be vegetarians because they have a lower rate of breast cancer. I'm simply saying that I think we need to get nutrition from various food products while we increase the consumption of fresh fruits, vegetables, and whole grains—and avoid obesity (that last one's a toughie that I'm still wrestling with). Whole-grain cereals (fruits and vegetables, too) are excellent sources of fiber and nutrition.

Make sure you're getting plenty of Vitamins A, C, and E in the daily diet. Whatever you do, don't overdose on vitamins in the form of tablets or capsules. Excessive amounts could be toxic. Instead, try to get vitamins in their natural form. Dark green and deep yellow vegetables (carrots, tomatoes, and spinach) and certain fruits (apricots, peaches, and cantaloupes) are rich in carotene, a form of Vitamin A, which is believed to lower the incidence of certain cancers (larynx, esophagus, and lung). Leafy vegetables, whole-grain cereals, nuts, and beans are good sources of Vitamin E. Ascorbic acid (Vitamin C) is found in citrus fruits, such as oranges. A well-balanced diet would have some Vitamin C in it. Of course, cabbage, broccoli, brussels sprout, cauliflower and other members of the "mustard family" (cruciferous vegetables) are all good for maintaining a balanced, nutrition-rich diet.

Until someone comes up with a cure for cancer, I think it's

only common sense to use every tool at our disposal, such as the American Cancer Society recommendations on diet and nutrition. The ACS also suggests that you leave the booze alone—as well as certain salt-cured and smoked meats. A phone call will get you all the pamphlets you want on the subject. I know some of these recommendations are controversial; that's why we have so many diet and health books on the market today.

What I've tried to do is cut through to the nitty-gritty. Follow a balanced diet of fruits, vegetables, whole grains, a little chicken (skinless) or fish, and maybe a good lean steak now and then. Cut out fatty foods, lay off the booze and chemicals and preservatives, and check the source of your foods as best you can. Take time to read the ingredient lists on all cans and packages; know what's in your foods.

I'm for Mama's food, all cleaned and healthy.

Now, let's get to the eating.

Ann loves to start the day with my Parade of Fruit, followed by a small bowl of special oatmeal. Let's talk oatmeal. I use the real stuff, old-fashion rolled oats; none of that instant junk for me. I pour pure mountain spring water in my pot, then add just the right amount of oats recommended on the box. Skip the salt, and no butter! My secret is to start the water and oats at the same time (most recipes call for adding oats to boiling water) as it makes the oats creamier-looking and tastier. Cook the oats on medium-high heat for five minutes or until the water is absorbed, stirring constantly or you'll burn the bottom of the pot. Then just before serving the oats, I stir in half a cup of skim milk (cuts fat to a minimum) and the oatmeal gets white and pretty. For a special taste, I add a little brown sugar on mine (it's a poor man's maple syrup) or a handful of raisins at the beginning makes a fine sweetener. Martha tells me she uses dietetic brown sugar because of Bob's diabetes. Ann mostly puts a few slices of banana left over from her Parade of Fruit. Some days I talk her into eating a slice of whole-grain bread with nuts. If Ann is on a diet (tell me when she isn't) I have to argue a bit to get her to eat the bread because she says it makes two starches—oatmeal and bread. She's right, so I never insist.

Other breakfasts include fresh juice and whole-grain bread with nuts (if she doesn't have oatmeal, then she has to eat the bread) or an egg every once in a while. Soft-boil the egg—no butter, no salt. I chop it up in a cup so it seems like a lot, and I break up a slice of whole-grain bread into little pieces dropping some into the egg to make it nice and chewy.

We try to eat our big meal in late afternoon and it is mostly salads. Be sure to make different ones, not the same one all the time or your customer might eat elsewhere. I do a lot with tuna (plain and no mayo), lettuce, tomatoes, and lots of onions sliced thin, but not too long.

To make salads tasty, I draw on my Spanish background to create a salsa sauce that Ann loves. You might want to give it a try.

ANDY'S SASSY SALSA SAUCE
(Serves four to six persons)

    4 medium tomatoes
    1 medium onion
    2 bunches cilantro
    Assorted chile peppers to suit your taste
    2 or more garlic cloves, to taste
    Juice of two lemons
    2 tablespoons tomato juice (optional)

Chop all ingredients into very small pieces and mix well—or combine in blender or food processor.

This is a good low-calorie salad dressing as well as a dip for tortilla chips. It can also be added to tacos or burritos or anything you want to flavor. Try it over some avocado slices. Talk about goooooooood. When Ann puts my tasty sauce on her salads, she smiles ear to ear. She knows I left out the fattening salad dressing in the colored bottles and I cut down on cholesterol, too. My salsa mix is not fattening, very low in calories. Make it fresh, though. It loses something in storage.

Another big favorite is my:

TURKEY BURRITO

3 pounds ground turkey (lean, no skin)
Kitchen Bouquet browning spray
1 onion, chopped
1 bunch cilantro
2 cans refried beans (no lard)
5 medium tomatoes, chopped
1 head lettuce, shredded
1 cup sour cream (we're being a little naughty here;
  substitute yoghurt if you want to reduce the calories)
2 cups mashed avocado
1 package of flour or corn tortillas (vegetarian type, no
  lard)
salsa
1 bag tortilla chips (no lard)

Spray turkey with Kitchen Bouquet browning spray, then stir-fry meat with onions. Add a little cilantro when meat is nearly finished. When meat is cooked, remove pan or wok from heat and cover until ready to serve. Heat refried beans. Have chopped tomatoes, shredded lettuce, sour cream, and avocado ready to serve in individual serving bowls. In non-stick skillet, heat tortillas over low heat just until hot and still soft. Place two tablespoons of refried beans (spread it around like peanut butter), then add about three tablespoons of the meat mixture and serve individually, allowing each person to "doctor" his or her own with the condiments of choice. V-8 vegetable juice with a celery stalk goes well with this. Serve with the salsa and tortilla chips on a nice summer day.

Some evenings we have sweet potatoes or white potatoes in their skins. No butter! After you get used to their good, sweet, natural taste you won't miss the butter. Along with a nice dinner salad, Ann can make a meal of either variety of potatoes with maybe steamed or raw carrots, which she likes sliced thin.

Ann's favorite dish is "Meat Loaf by André" (it's got to have a fancy title), which is made with turkey. This dish always makes her suspicious. When she gets this, she knows I want something.

MEAT LOAF BY ANDRÉ
(That's me, Andy)

> 2 *pounds extra lean ground turkey meat sprayed with*
> *Kitchen Bouquet (you can use lean beef if you insist)*
> 2 *eggs*
> 1–2 *teaspoons salt (if you must!)*
> 1 *15-ounce can 100 percent natural tomato soup*
> 1 *cup finely grated whole-grain bread with nuts*
> 1 *clove garlic*
> 5 *tablespoons chopped onion*
> 1 *cup grated Italian cheese (I mix several types but they*
> *are all Italian imports)*

Mix all ingredients by hand in a big bowl. Pack the mixture into a *slightly* oiled (vegetable oil) nine-inch-loaf glass baking dish. Cook at 350–375 degrees F for one hour. Test for doneness; cook for fifteen minutes if it is not done enough for you, but don't overcook. Make sure you see the great-tasting juice in the loaf dish bubbling. This juice keeps the loaf from winding up dry like some meat loafs. Not mine!

To complete the meal, toss a small salad or serve a vegetable of your choice.

And now for dessert.

BANANA PINEAPPLE PSEUDO ICE CREAM

Peel and freeze one banana per person and two strips of pineapple per person. Just before serving, place frozen fruits in a powerful juicer, blender, or food processor (if your machine is not powerful enough, it won't be able to handle the frozen fruit). Mix until the fruit is the consistency of ice cream. You can choose your own fruits, but always use a frozen banana because it gives the dessert its consistency. If the mixture is too thick, add a *tiny bit* of fruit juice to the juicer, blender, or food processor.

There are many recipes for good, smart eating. If you don't know where to start, sit down or, better yet, take a walk with your wife through the supermarket. Bring a notepad and ask her what she likes in each category (cereals, noodles, citrus fruits, green vegetables, dairy products, meats, etc.) Then, on your own, learn what's healthiest for her of the foods she likes. Make a second, permanent list of these foods and search for recipes that incorporate them. You'll soon have a collection of healthy favorites.

And, finally, a few ideas on how to keep the munchies at bay. We keep fresh fruit—some cold and some at room temperature—throughout the house. Fruit makes a snack that is filling and good for you. We also keep a good supply of popcorn—easy on the salt and *no* butter allowed.

Also banned from our house are ice cream (Ann's favorite), nondiet sodas, chips, and greasy fried foods. We know it's difficult, but if it's not in the house, you're not going to eat it. The key is good food in moderation; don't overdo any of them.

I know you're wondering if Ann Jillian ever cheats on her diet? Does Andy ever help her?

You bet we do! But in very small quantities and not too often. Ice cream is Ann's favorite—especially vanilla. The key is to treat yourself and not fall off the good food wagon.

10

Building Your Wife's Support System

Without exception, the medical professionals we have dealt with believe that a strong support system is an extremely important factor in improving a cancer patient's chances for survival. The key is the support offered by family and friends. And it makes sense. If everyone is pulling for your wife, it can't help but encourage her to fight.

A cancer patient needs the constant reassurance and loving support that come from a nurturing family and close friends. She should be left alone as little as possible, especially during those difficult days following hospitalization or treatment. She is often too weak to care for herself or too depressed to keep up her spirits.

If possible, make sure that your wife does not have to go by herself for appointments or treatments. You may not be able to be with her during some of the actual treatments, but she knows you are there. If you can't make it, then arrange for someone—one of your children, a member of your family, or a friend—to go with her. This may require a bit of sacrifice on your part, but it can be done.

Don't be afraid to ask for help if you need it. Too often,

people stand ready to help but don't know what to do or even that you need help.

Bob: I decided that it would be easier for the doctors to check the progress of Martha's healing if her pajamas were split along the seam on the left side and then refastened with Velcro. This would allow her to wear pajamas and rid herself of those unsightly hospital gowns while allowing the doctor free access to her incision.

I turned to Delilah Perkins, age ninety-two, for help. It was her aged hands that ripped the seams and hand-stitched the Velcro in place. She was delighted to be of help.

Delilah also called Martha at least twice a week. The spunk of that aged lady refreshed Martha's spirits.

Concern came from every direction. Martha returned from the hospital to a sparkling house courtesy of her children. They had even gotten the curtains cleaned to protect her from germs since chemotherapy inhibits the immune system. Our kitchen table overflowed with food cooked by ladies of the church.

Several days later, a neighbor came over with a complete meal—including dessert—and stored it in the refrigerator.

Cards poured in, friends and neighbors dropped by with inspirational books. Flower arrangements dotted the house. Everyone took particular joy in a glowing summer bouquet from Ann and Andy.

If you are members of a church or synagogue, you can find untold help from fellow members. Besides helping with meals and cleaning the house, they will assist with hospital visitors, volunteer to baby-sit, drive patients to treatments, etc. A number of churches have day-care centers that are excellent for smaller children. It has been our experience that help is always available if you seek it. A minister told us that such an organized effort also helps your friends because being helpful gives *them* a way of expressing their support for such a seriously ill friend.

You haven't been to church or synagogue in years, what do you do? A number of the larger churches have counselors on staff—not just as an evangelical tool, but to help people experiencing tough times. Once contacted, they can put you in touch with members of the congregation who have already been through your trials. This can ease your reentry into things religious, if that's what you seek, or give you the help you need, if that's what you seek, or both. Pick up the telephone and tap in—these people are ready to help.

Social organizations and friends often go untapped because "I don't want to be a bother." It's worth exploring. Many city service clubs (are you a member of one?) have committees to help in times of illness by providing food and transportation. We have found that friends are quick to volunteer help (how many times have you sincerely offered to help but never received a call?) but don't know what else to do unless you let them know what is needed. They may not push their help on you because they don't want to intrude. Also contact the American Cancer Society for a list of support organizations. The hospital where you wife was treated or the radiation center or oncology center will probably have such an organization.

Ann and Andy also received support in the form of cards and letters from people they had never met before—Ann's devoted fans.

Andy: When the news broke that Ann Jillian had breast cancer and that both of her breasts were to be removed to save her life, we experienced an outpouring of love that defies description. Within a month, more than forty thousand pieces of mail arrived at our home as loving support flowed in from complete strangers. Actually, they weren't complete strangers. Ann visited these folks every week when she came into their homes through the modern miracle of television.

From the tone and volume of mail, it was obvious that she was known to them and that they liked her a lot. Some even loved her a lot. They sent prayer cards by the hundreds, from

every possible faith you could think of. One especially loving couple even took time from their vacation to send a note:

"Please know that our hearts go out to you and your husband as you fight breast cancer. We were on vacation in Israel when we heard the news and we purchased a tree for you there. It was planted in your name in Israel because just as Israel is and the Jewish people are survivors, we feel that you too are a survivor and you will be well soon. God bless you."

Ann hopes to see that tree one day.

People reached out to say, "We feel for you. We are concerned" in so many ways.

We received many thousands of letters and notes and cards. One letter with a simple message illustrates the thousands:

"For all the hours of enjoyment you have given me and my family, I want you to know that we are pulling for you and love you in a special way although we have never met.

"You are like a member of our family and we cried when we heard you were ill and we will keep you in our prayers for a complete recovery."

Another group of people also responded: those whose lives have been touched by cancer, either breast or another cancer. We heard from victims and family members of victims. The expertise they passed along to Ann and me was invaluable. Thousands of people sat down and wrote their hearts out. They had this old cop crying on so many occasions that I lost count. You have to realize that most of my life, all I ever really saw was the underbelly of our society and the cruel acts some people perpetrated on each other. As I watched this love pour in, and contrasted it to my previous experience on the vice beat, it taught me a lesson in life that I will never forget.

In time I would see more than a hundred thousand pieces of mail from loving people who cared about another member of the human race who was suffering through an ordeal. They saw the way Ann was trying to get back up and into life so fast. They applauded that in her. It was as if they were standing by her bedside rooting their heads off for her and this was the best medicine.

Those hundred thousand pieces of mail said that the people were more than willing to accept Ann back as an entertainer. You see, their love was getting stronger just like mine and Ann's! The people cared and Ann has often told me:

"I only wish that every person who ever had breast cancer could experience the strength taken from all this mail, from these 'lovers of life' out there. They will never know how much easier it was for me to recover because of this mail and the love it contained."

It's a shame that everyone does not have the opportunity to experience a similar outpouring of support the way Ann has. Regrettably, there is no way the media can tell us that Martha Stewart or any other woman is suffering from breast cancer so we could all get behind her and give her the loving support and love that everyone should have.

Ann is determined to respond to all mail with a return address. She still handles about twenty letters of thanks per week. We have large boxes we work from in storage. We try to answer it all in the order in which it was opened, but we admit that we give special consideration to the ladies who have gone through breast cancer and I take a special interest in the many loving husbands who write.

11

Life Without Breasts

Let's face a reality that we all have to deal with now that the crisis is over. It's possible that your wife no longer has breasts or that she has only one. How do you feel about this? In a follow-up letter to the conversation that launched this book, Andy wrote, "I would like to know if feelings that I have are the same as others, or am I on my own here? There are so many thoughts that must be dealt with. What do we do when some woman walks past who is obviously well endowed? Do we look? Do we stare at the tops of our shoes?"

It's a valid concern. After months of battling to keep our wives physically and emotionally intact, we wouldn't want this problem to harm—or possibly destroy—what has been achieved. We believe that the answer will have to be worked out in an open and honest way between you and your wife.

A survey by the American Institute of Cancer Research revealed that men had similar anxieties and feelings about the loss of a breast as women. Eighty-one percent of those surveyed said that if they faced the prospect of a wife or partner losing a breast, they would feel compassion and support. They further stated that their expressions of love would be no different after mastectomy.

One oncologist told us that men get a bum rap, that the majority are helpful and supportive of their wife or lover. But a diagnosis of breast cancer still presents a crisis in most marriages. The degree of this crisis will depend on the maturity of the individuals and the maturity of their relationship. This is going to be a stressful time that requires two-way communication. The crisis you face now is not unlike that of shared grief at the death of a loved one. You both will experience some of the emotions of grief, so share the loss. If your wife tries to talk to you about her loss, don't dismiss her with the easy answer, "It doesn't make any difference to me." Sure it makes a difference, to both of you. She is going to or already has lost a part of her body; you have seen a loved one suffer and she is no longer exactly as she was. A breast is one symbol of her femininity; its loss makes a difference to *both* of you. Recognize what you are both experiencing.

We believe there is also great truth in the counseling offered by one minister in sessions with parishioners about to marry. He warns them that sex is twenty percent of a good marriage and ninety percent of a bad marriage. So, if you have a marginal marriage, something like a major illness—especially one with as drastic a consequence as a mastectomy— can be exceedingly stressful. If a marriage is tottering because sex is its main element, then this illness could push it over the brink; but it doesn't have to. The tendency is to consider the husband the culprit in such a scenario, but the wife could be just as guilty by becoming consumed by the loss of her breast and withdrawing from her husband. These can be trying times, but remember that any problem can be worked out by a couple willing to invest the patience, kindness, and love it takes to help each other.

Marth's oncologist believes "The man can get a raw deal. Sometimes he comes in for unjust criticism or generalized blame. I can recall only one time that a divorce occurred because of a mastectomy." Ann and Andy have talked to hundreds of couples, and instances of marriage breakups because of breast cancer appear to be in the overwhelming minority.

There are some caveats men should observe. For instance, it would be only natural for your wife to become jealous if you stared at a buxom woman like you'd never seen a female before. After all, we do live in a breast-conscious society and that will place an added strain on your wife. It is up to you to convince her that your love is encompassed in her very existence—the sum total of her being. It was never solely in her parts.

We suggest having a candid discussion with your wife. You might be surprised at her reaction if you frankly admit that you miss her breasts. She can understand that. She misses them, too. It can be a shared loss instead of each of you harboring your own grief.

You are only human. God created you with certain desires and the flash of a breast could kindle them. Remember that oldie but goodie, a rock ditty entitled "Poison Ivy"? One of the verses goes, "You can look, but you'd better not touch."

We really doubt that fidelity will be a problem for most men. It's inconceivable to us that a man would jeopardize his future happiness with a woman he has fought so hard to keep by his side. But we are not foolish enough to believe it can't happen, so we encourage continued self-discipline; if you're happily married, then you are already disciplined. If you don't have self-discipline, then try it, you might like it. And it might not hurt at this point to reread the "Steps to Maturity" in Chapter One.

Also, don't let this hamper your sex life. It can be just as fulfilling as before. There may be problems such as early onset of menopause, which is often brought on by chemotherapy. Menopause may rob a woman of natural secretions, causing vaginal dryness, which can lead to pain during intercourse. Chemotherapy may force you to postpone your sex life for a few months but you'll survive.

Don't be afraid to talk to a doctor about this. He or she will give you a number of practical guidelines to overcome the physical discomfort associated with menopause. Be sure to discuss any marital aids you use with the oncologist. He may caution against certain creams, lubricants, and drugs that might affect your wife's hormonal balance. Before the discussion, ask your wife if she would prefer that you speak alone to the doctor or if she wants to participate. We know that it shouldn't make any difference—a doctor's a doctor—but the sex of the physician might make a difference to her. Either way, the two of you should prepare a list of questions that you both want asked. That way she can still have input should she decline at the last minute.

You may have psychological problems. The surgery may affect your romantic feelings to the extent that your sexual drive is lessened. If this happens, we suggest you seek professional help. Don't let macho stand in your way or make you feel guilty about needing advice. A few sessions may help you work your way through your problem. Remember, no two people go through an experience in the same way. Your reaction is uniquely yours.

The way we look at it is that we are two loving and devoted husbands. Neither of us plans on having mistresses or being unfaithful, ever. That means that we face the rest of our lives without breast contact. While we don't like it, it seems like a small price to pay when we think of Ann's and Martha's sacrifices.

And more than anything else, we have the women we love by our sides.

Andy: I have noticed from all the letters I've received that this is a serious consequence that men have to come to terms with. Now that our wives are out of danger, it may even seem a bit selfish to consider it. But we must.

The idea of going through life without ever having the pleasure of my wife's breasts seemed like a raw deal to me. I didn't feel this way until a long time after Ann was on her way to recovery. But the thought did occur to me and I have to deal with it.

It is very easy to state what is obviously important. I have my wife, alive, and with me. That's what I want. But it is a little

more difficult to cope with underlying emotions that surface from time to time. To say I would not want my wife's breasts back would be a lie. I do wish them back. I wish I could wave my hand and undo all that has happened; that Ann would have her breasts and never have had cancer. But it did happen and her breasts are gone, no matter how hard I wish otherwise.

How do I feel about it? In all honesty, I miss them very much, very often; but not enough to get carried away about it.

I was always a bigger "heart" man anyway. My lovely wife still has her bigger-than-life heart. To me, a lady with a heart, who really cared for others—and could show it—was a lady who always caught my eye. A woman could have the best pair going, but if that's all she had, she didn't have me for long.

On a physical level, I was always attracted to a lady's face. If she had a cute face, then I was that much more attracted to her. It was a combination of face and heart that helped me decide whether to explore a deeper relationship.

When I met Ann, I quickly found out that she was not the run-of-the-mill Hollywood cutie. She had brains, personality, and charm. Her Old World upbringing appealed to me a great deal.

It was Ann's face, not her breasts, that first caught my attention. That oh-so-wonderful face captured me so completely, it was several days before I checked out the rest of her.

You bet she had breasts. I found them the most beautiful this old copper'd ever laid eyes on. But after the face and heart, I'm a butt and leg man. Actually, I'm the type of guy who could always find something attractive about any woman.

As you can see, breasts were never at the top of my list. My Ann may not have her breasts, but she has all I will ever need in my life from a wife. We both get sad from time to time that her breasts are gone, but we quickly count our blessings and we know darn well we can—and will—live without them. She certainly couldn't live *with* them.

This may not be as easy for you as it is for me. Each man is different. But it is a relatively small price to pay for our lover to be alive and well.

A suggestion: Rediscover kissing her great lips! That should give you the oral pleasure you need. Since the surgery, Ann and I are kissing fools. We have discovered a silver-lining and rediscovered our youth. Sometimes we feel just like a teenage couple at our first dance, experiencing their first kiss.

What I'm trying to get across here is that it's okay to miss your wife's breasts. Some of us will miss them more than others. But there are other compensations—none more pleasurable than the sight of your wife laughing, happy, alive, content, and secure in your love.

And finally, this reaction from Ann.

After Ann's surgery, as a good husband, I was not about to even glance in the direction of a woman who walked by who had obviously been blessed with a great pair of breasts. I would turn my head, or do an about-face if she was walking toward me, and other silly things to avoid having to look at her. I didn't want Ann to see me look because I felt this would make her feel bad or think I was desirous of a woman with breasts. This could not have been further from the truth.

One day Annie saw my pattern and said to me:

"Hey, lover man, breasts are things of beauty. God gave you eyes so you can look. So look. Don't gawk. But take a look if they are worth looking at. Don't stare. Don't make a fool of yourself. Do as you did before. Whatever you did then is okay now."

I told her about my fear of hurting her. She took my hand and reassured me, "No way!"

We hugged, and what relief I felt, thanks to Ann.

It should be pointed out that there are problems unique to couples where the wife has lost one breast as compared to couples who face an immediate double mastectomy. The two mastectomies may be separated by days, months, or even years and there is the subconscious tension of "waiting for the other shoe to drop" no matter how often you tell yourself that it won't.

While a single mastectomy may help a woman retain a

heightened sense of femininity, it can create a problem for the husband. What does he do? How does he pursue the pleasure of sex in this situation? We believe it is best to have a frank discussion with your wife in which you establish boundaries for mutual enjoyment. Open communication should never harm anyone.

Bob: I faced a slightly different set of problems from Andy. Martha lost each breast a year apart. Because of the nature of the cancerous tumor, and its size, we were in the unique position of praying that the chemotherapy and radiation would work and that Martha would have the opportunity to have a life-saving mastectomy.

It was a year of peaks and valleys until the doctors said that clinical evaluation could find no trace of cancer. Then it was our decision. As you know, we opted for the surgery as insurance. It's possible that I wanted the mastectomy more than Martha because it would tell us her medical condition.

Therefore, aside from the obvious emotions, it wasn't too traumatic to lose the first breast because we had prayed long and hard to be in a position just to have the surgery.

A year later, a questionable mass appeared in the other breast and a biopsy was ordered. It wasn't cancer, but this time it was Martha who pushed for the mastectomy because she didn't want to go through a series of biopsies over the years.

Because of her situation, I had a year of transition between the first and second mastectomy. I doubt it made things any easier. At times the single breast seemed to interfere with our relationship. I was often hesitant to touch it because I was fearful it would remind Martha of her loss. When I broached the subject, she reassured me that it didn't.

The days leading up to the second mastectomy were ones of turmoil. Fears about touching the remaining breast resurfaced. Should I talk to her about the pending surgery? I elected to keep my hands to myself and do a lot of positive talking and reassuring. I also felt it would be morbid to heighten our awareness of the single breast that would soon be gone. I know I've pushed throughout this book for open, honest discussion, but in this case I felt it was best to keep my own counsel about our sex life and her breast and not discuss the situation other than in terms of the loss of her remaining breast. Since the second mastectomy we've had many talks about our sex life.

I know it's corny but I tell Martha that each surgical scar is a beauty mark. At least they are beautiful to me because without them, I wouldn't have her and her beauty is so much more than merely physical. And in my eyes, she is still that beautiful, graceful, long-haired young girl who elected to share her love with me more than a quarter century ago. The trauma she has had to suffer in losing her breasts has only heightened my love and devotion to her. And she certainly hasn't lost her sex appeal to me.

"How could you think I'm beautiful?" she'll scoff sometimes. "I'm a mass of scars and I've gained weight."

"Of course, I'm Robert Redford," is my reply, which causes her to smile, because if there is one thing I'm not, it's a handsome, athletic specimen. "Let's keep it in perspective. I want you. I don't want anything or anyone else. I'm so thankful to have you that nothing else matters."

Sure, I miss her breasts. Especially at the times we are alone and she's standing with her back to me. Unconsciously I walk up behind her and sneak my arms around her in a caressing motion, something I've done thousands of times. Because it is an unconscious, natural reflex, it both pleases and perplexes her.

"You forget they're not there," she says before I realize that she's right. I just didn't think about it. Then I'm perplexed and pleased. I must not miss them or I wouldn't do that; but then again, maybe I do long to caress them or I wouldn't do that; or maybe I'm just the most forgetful person in the world.

I know that I had trouble remembering which breast was removed first. Sometimes I would have to visualize her lying in the hospital bed and which side the bandages were on so I could remember.

And, men, you have to be careful of those "realistic" pros-
theses. On several occasions, and to Martha's amusement, I
found I'd been having a cheap thrill because I wasn't caressing
the real thing. True story. Really happened!

Men, put yourself in her position. Wouldn't you hate to
think that you could have surgery that would drive your wife
away from you; that she couldn't love you because of some-
thing completely out of your control? Fortunately, most people
are bigger than that.

And the truth of it is that breasts are not what makes a
woman sexy. It's what is happening in her mind that makes her
sexy. A sexy woman just is. It is not any one part of her, but
it is all *of her. Sexiness is also part of her own self-image. If*
she feels sexy, then we perceive her as sexy.

A man's breasts do not have the same significance, so it
is difficult to imagine a woman's emotional state at this time.
Her fear of death is compounded by her potential loss of a
positive self-image and her fear of losing sex appeal in your
eyes.

And, finally, what about the single woman and the man or
men in her life?

She faces a unique situation that we know is filled with
anguish and uncertainty. The single women we talked with all
expressed the same fears experienced by a married woman:
first the fear of dying, then the fear of loss of sexual attractiveness. But their stress was compounded by the question, "Will
a man love me now?" One woman put it this way:

"About a year before my cancer I went through a terrible
divorce. After the diagnosis I wondered what would happen to
me. If I had been married, I would already have had someone
and we could have adjusted and gone through this together.
Now, anyone I met would have to accept me as I am. I didn't
know if there would be anyone out there like that."

There was. A year later she met a man who loved her for
herself and they are now happily married.

You can understand her fears. She questioned herself.

What would she bring to this relationship that could lead to marriage?

This is a tough reality to face; but it can be faced and conquered.

In a support group meeting, a vivacious young lady recalled meeting a man at her apartment complex. After a period of time passed, they were swimming when she decided it would be best to tell him about her surgery.

"He said, 'Well, if you only have one, we'll have to take especially good care of it,' " she recalled with a grin. "I thought, 'What a special guy.' "

With or without breasts, there are special people in this world—both male and female. And sometimes that special guy doesn't have to be someone interested in her sexually. Many breast cancer victims discover the need to talk to a man, especially women without a husband or fiancé, to explore the masculine point-of-view. One young woman uncovered new depths in her father when she turned to him for supportive and open discussions on this topic. This special father reassured his daughter, who at thirty-eight was consumed with fears, and helped bridge the gap until she could regain her own self-assurance.

12

Man to Man

From time to time a husband should take a minute to stop and ask the question, "How am I doing?"

This book has centered on your wife and what you can do to support her as she copes with breast cancer. But you are in the battle, too, and occasionally you need to take a few minutes for yourself. Your emotions are being buffeted and you need to understand both yourself and your situation.

This is a crucial time in your life. If you find yourself confused, scared, full of indecision, and fearful of your wife's possible death, then your reactions are more or less normal. To a lesser degree, you will find yourself fighting the same dual battle as your wife: mental and physical. It is important to take a few minutes for self-evaluation, so spend some private time considering your own physical and mental state.

Take a break. No, we don't mean running off with the boys to play poker and drink beer or taking an extended fishing trip. We mean something that is both mentally and physically refreshing. We didn't know how to take a break. If there had been a magic button to press for a few hours relief, it would have been Godsent. Now we understand the importance of physical activity in relaxing both the body and the mind. You might try golf or tennis or swimming or racquetball. You might get out in the yard with your children and kick a football or pitch a baseball. Any type of physical activity will help relieve your mind and ease physical tension. If it's summer, work up a big sweat in your yard—that will do both you and the yard some good. If it's winter, go to the shopping mall and walk briskly around; some malls even have quarter-mile markers to help you keep track of the distance. A couple of brisk miles will wipe the cobwebs from your mind. The exercise will keep you strong and you need to stay physically fit to be in shape to better help your wife.

Bob: My problems were compounded by the fact that the week following the discovery of Martha's cancer, I was diagnosed as being diabetic. It wasn't particularly a shock since the majority of my family has the disease. The doctors believe the combination of family history, being overweight, and the emotional shock of Martha's illness possibly pushed me over the edge.

The family doctor put me on medication and a strict diet. After a year I was able to control it by diet and weight loss.

Our dental student son had this wry observation.

"We now have two of the top three killers in America in our family."

Work out your feelings, so that you'll be in control of your emotions. We both feel our visits to a psychiatrist did us a lot of good, especially in helping to control our own emotional state. If you have even the slightest suspicion that it would help, then try at least one visit. If you can't afford a psychiatrist, then go to a qualified psychologist or talk to your clergyman.

If you feel so low that you just want to sit down and cry, then go ahead, it won't hurt. It is nature's way of relieving tension. You might even get your best buddy and cry on his shoulder. It worked for us.

Andy: I have always been a take-charge guy, so it was a new experience for me when I found myself in need of comfort. Some mornings, especially right after the diagnosis when my emotions were particularly raw, I would wake up before Annie and sneak out to the guest house to talk to my sister and her husband.

The truth of the matter is, I had a good cry.

Other times I would call Bob and we'd comfort each other. Then I'd wash my face, strap on a smile that said everything was going to be all right, and go back to my Annie.

Those private times helped me make it. I needed to have a release and I strongly suggest you consider finding a friend who can act as your safety valve.

You also have to keep a close watch on yourself, because you're going to experience emotions and thoughts that will be new to you. Sometimes your mind will drift into painful areas, but even that can be helpful, as one way to confront pain and unpleasantness is to think your way through it.

You might even find your subconscious at work in unique and revealing ways.

Bob: I'm not normally a dreamer, but I've had a couple of interesting ones since this started. The first occurred shortly after we discovered Martha had cancer.

I dreamed that a burglar had entered the house and attacked Martha. What followed was a battle to end all battles as the burglar and I fought throughout the darkened house, demolishing every room. It seemed that he was always just a few inches from grabbing Martha and I had never felt so desperate. I awoke breathing hard, my heart pounding, and, yes, just like in the movies, I was sweating profusely.

The next day, when I told Martha about it, she asked if the burglar ever got her.

"No," I said and she smiled.

Like myself, she had surmised that the dream-burglar

represented her cancer. A psychiatrist later confirmed our analysis.

The other dream occurred just a few days before her second mastectomy. I don't know how many times I prayed that any recurrence of the disease be visited on me. I believe the second dream had something to do with that desire.

I dreamed that killer bees swarmed around the two of us and fortunately, I attracted them away from her and they all landed on me, covering my groin area.

There was no pain, and as can only happen in a dream, the bees were all under my clothing where they couldn't be seen, but became a pulsating mass that turned into honeycombs. I reached down and used my hands to pop the honeycomb and the bees through my clothing, killing them all. Again she was saved from harm.

The comforting message of these two dreams was the fact that I always won and that my wife was always safe.

And, finally, we challenge you to "hunker down."

Anyone who's ever been in a shooting war knows what it means to hunker down. A soldier on the battlefields of Europe or Korea or in the jungles of Vietnam understands what it means to hunker down so small that you can practically hide behind a blade of grass. It's a good, down-home term that describes the ability to have staying power no matter what the circumstances or the dangers.

Now it's time to hunker down against cancer. This could be the most difficult challenge of all because life will be constantly changing as new values surface to put a new focus on your life.

You need to hunker down for the short term (for the immediate battle) and for the long term (the months and years as you learn to live with the constant threat that cancer may return). This positive, stoic stance will keep you strong in a hurricane of emotions. From time to time you might find yourself again experiencing rage at the situation or impatience at the progress of treatment, or being angry at the world, or questioning "Why her?" and "Why me?" or bargaining with God or simply feeling frustration. Expect this to happen and don't be discouraged.

At the top of this chapter we asked you to consider, "How am I doing?"

If you've gone through most of these emotions, or are still going through them (you might experience them singularly, in pairs, or all at one time), and if you haven't let them keep you from acting, then we'll answer for you. We believe you're doing fine.

Hunker down and fight by taking action. Action helps ease tension and stress and puts you on the road to survival. But don't be surprised if all of the above emotions recur as you face new problems.

But now you will be better prepared to continue because experience counts. Each day will get a little easier for you to help your wife and yourself at the same time. Experience will help ease the burden of stress and anxiety.

So hunker down and hang tough.

_13_

Give of Yourself

We ask that you give of yourself as another way to fight back.

Ann and Andy have spent untold hours attending seminars and clinics, making speeches and public appearances to spread the message that you _can_ fight back.

Ann has been in the forefront of this battle.

"It has been proven that when anyone in the public eye is stricken with something, it saves lives," Ann said when it was announced that First Lady Nancy Reagan would have a mastectomy. At the time Ann was filming _The Ann Jillian Story,_ a telemovie focusing on her courtship and marriage to Andy and their battle with breast cancer. Ann immediately sent a telegram of support, remembering all the letters of support she received. As he watched his wife lead the cast and crew in prayers for the First Lady's safe recovery, Andy couldn't help but recall the time Ann met President Ronald Reagan.

Andy: After her surgery, Ann was offered every type of award there is. She appreciated them all, but one was rather special because it came from a fellow cancer patient and thespian.

She received the American Cancer Society's Courage Award, presented by President Ronald Reagan in the Oval Office on March 25, 1986.

When he read the award and emphasized that Ann was being honored for helping to teach the nation about the "hopeful" side of breast cancer, we all knew what he meant; Ann has spoken to so many groups, made so many one-on-one phone calls to other women having a bad time, and answered so much mail. Ann has something akin to a ministry in her letters and phone calls. Her work fighting cancer has curtailed her personal time, time she would like to spend with her family and working on her entertainment career.

As she accepted the award from the President, she said: "On behalf of all the women and their families and for all people who have had their lives touched by cancer, I accept this for *them!*"

To us, the President was a "sample copy" of the loving people who wrote to us by the thousands. Neither Ann nor I will ever forget that day in the White House. We knew he understood.

We only wish that every other lady or man who has had to face cancer could have seen the love and compassion in the President's eyes that day.

When the President praised Ann's battle, she noted: "All I did was what you did—brush myself off and get back to work."

"Yes, but you look much better than I ever looked on camera," he said with a laugh.

Ann replied, "That was so sweet. Can I give you a kiss? Is it okay?"

"Is it okay?" the President asked, looking around. "It's okay with me."

And she planted one on his cheek! He laughed and the others present laughed, too. Little did we know that his family, too, would soon face the battle against breast cancer. None of us ever know.

As time goes by, Ann finds herself more and more able to resume her career, giving fewer interviews on her battle with breast cancer. She now declines media interviews about her personal struggle (numerous magazine and newspaper articles have been written, her movie has aired), preferring to tell her story at private lectures she makes to groups of people invited to hear her speak. Of course, she is always open to help with other breast cancer-related venues, such as fund raisers, etc. She will never quit working for the well-being of cancer victims and promoting early detection through her work with the American Cancer Society.

Ann and Andy have added five letters to their "You've saved my life file" since *The Ann Jillian Story* aired. Each letter is a documented case of a woman whose life was saved after she read an article or saw Ann on television and was inspired to get a checkup that revealed breast cancer and thereby saved her life. The movie was the number-one two-hour movie on television for the 1987–88 season, including all three networks. It scored higher than any other telemovie or feature movie. Except for one, it also outscored all the very expensive network miniseries.

Ann's work was also honored by her peers. *The Ann Jillian Story* brought with it the Emmy nomination for Ann in the outstanding lead-actress category; the movie itself being nominated for an Emmy as outstanding drama/comedy special.

But your wife doesn't have to be an Ann Jillian to save lives. While Ann has touched thousands of lives, Martha has played a key role in the lives of her friends. Sometimes there's not a lot you can do, but cards, meals, and a telephone call of "courage!" help people through the troubled times.

Warn your neighbors. Warn your friends. Encourage them to get checkups. And then stand by them when they're assailed by doubts and fears.

Bob: *As this book was being written, Martha got a frantic call one Saturday afternoon. It was Cindy Wulf, the family friend our daughter turned to the night we found her missing* *from the house. With Martha's surgery fresh in mind, Cindy took swift action that year when she discovered a lump in her breast. She had a mastectomy. But within months hepatitis struck her and that disease wouldn't respond properly to treatment.*

Based on her history, one doctor suggested a liver biopsy to determine exactly what drug was needed to treat the hepatitis. Then the doctor told her:

"There is the very slight possibility of a rare liver cancer that doesn't show up on X rays. I'm sure it's not that but we better check."

All Cindy heard were the words "liver cancer." It was the worst-case scenario in action. Although she had already been through the trauma of a breast cancer diagnosis, the words evoked a near-paralyzing fear; and we understood how she felt.

Cindy was terrified although the doctors had sought to reassure her. Martha went over and the two women had an afternoon-long coffee klatsch.

"It sounds to me like the doctors are just being careful," Martha told her. "And you want them to be careful. Besides, they told you they wanted to check your liver to find out what drug would be the most effective. She said that liver cancer was a rare possibility."

"But what if it's not?" was Cindy's anguished reply.

"Let's wait and see," Martha said. Then using a technique we had employed many times before, Martha began to make a list of all the reasons it should be all right. She then made a list of all the reasons it wouldn't be all right. The good list far outnumbered the bad. I stopped by and we all clasped hands in friendship and prayed.

Martha spent several more hours with Cindy on Sunday and we rejoiced with her Monday morning bright and early when the biopsy showed no sign of cancer.

A few days later, Martha received a beautiful card from Cindy with a written message that brought tears of joy to our eyes and our hearts.

I doubt Martha will ever be involved in any organized efforts to help others—that's just not her style. But she's beautiful to watch in a one-on-one.

And believe us, there is nothing more satisfying than knowing that you helped someone. Ann has received thousands of letters from women who conquered their fears and went to the doctor after putting off that first checkup.

Ann has often said that there is nothing she can do in her show business career that could ever come close to giving her the good feeling she gets when she reads one of these letters.

You will also discover that by being involved with others, you will have less time to worry about yourself as you are out there punching and doing your best to knock out cancer. It will give you a way of getting back at cancer and allow you to positively direct your anger. It may also give your wife the sense that something good has come from her struggle, that she can use it to help others.

Recall how you felt the first time you met someone who had already been through this ordeal and come through it successfully. You looked at them, you touched them, and you realized that it can be done.

One husband told us that words of wisdom and encouragement mean far more when they come from a former breast cancer patient—or her husband.

Share that special feeling.

Epilogue

We wanted a big finish for this book. We wanted to go out with the sun shining, bells ringing, bands playing, and flags waving, in fine theatrical style.

But then we realized that life isn't like the big production number that wraps up everything before the curtain call.

In real life, actors move on to a new role, musicians tune up for another performance, and sets are struck for the next play. That play is over—it's time to move on to the next performance.

And now is the time to move forward with your life. There will be good days when life is a glorious stage production and you proudly march at the head of the parade. There will also be days when it rains on your parade.

But we believe you now will see life with a perspective you've never experienced. We believe you will stop to smell the roses and exalt in the beauty of nature and ponder the wonder of human relationships. We believe you'll do this every day, because you never know what the next will bring, and each day is too precious to waste. As you experience the good

and the bad, as you practice faith, hope, and love, we believe
you will reach out and hold the hand of the woman you love.
After all, speaking man to man, what else is there?

Appendix:

Woman to Woman

QUESTIONS MOST FREQUENTLY ASKED OF ANN AND MARTHA

1. Were you afraid you would die?

Martha: Yes. Absolutely! I was terrified. Like many others, I translated the word "cancer" as "death." That is, I *did;* please note that is past tense. Now I don't, of course. I still view it as the killer disease it *can* be, but I know now that it does not *always* mean death.

It was obvious that my doctors believed the chances were slim that I would survive this horrible disease. Some voiced that belief, while it was evident in the expressions and attitudes of others. I knew the situation was grim. One doctor gave me a twenty percent chance of five-year survival—some said forty percent (I got several opinions) but none said more than forty percent. One, when pinned down, said less than fifty percent, but I put the words in his mouth. These are not very good odds. If your odds are not good, then forget them; we can beat odds. If odds couldn't be beaten, then I wouldn't be here to tell you this. On the other hand, if your odds sound good, by all means keep them in mind because you need all the encouragement you can get.

Ann: At first, no. A member of my family had overcome breast cancer more than thirty years ago, and today she is an active and healthy lady of eighty-one. I looked at her and did not fear dying. But when people started looking at me with a funny expression, like they

185

were thinking, "Oh, this is what they look like before they say the big good-bye," I got scared and realized that it was possible that this could kill me.

But with each passing day I was able to push the idea of dying to the back of my mind, especially when the lab report showed that the cancer had not spread to my lymph nodes.

Sure I'm fearful each time I go for a checkup, but each time I leave, it is with a clean bill of health. I feel that life is mine. Time has a way of easing a lot of things, including fear.

2. *Were you fearful that the loss of your breasts might possibly hurt your marriage?*

Ann: Yes. I was very concerned about Andy's feelings and how my surgery would affect our relationship. But this was soon dispelled by Andy's loving actions toward me. He showed me that our love was strong enough to withstand this physical loss.

Martha: No, absolutely not. I am one of the fortunate few who has a totally secure marriage. I can say that even more assuredly now than before the breast cancer because if this terrible ordeal couldn't rock our marriage, not much can. I'm not speaking only of the loss of breasts, but of cancer's entire emotional and physical spectrum.

I know that my body is not as appealing as it used to be, but that is not only because of the loss of breasts. We all get older even if we take great care of our bodies. Nobody can have an eighteen-year-old body forever. Not everyone loses breasts, but everyone gets older—if they're lucky enough to hang around long enough.

The inside of us (our character and soul) can remain beautiful, and even *improve.* Bob knows this and always points out the good things. We try to dwell on what we *do* have and not what we don't have, including breasts. I didn't loose *all* my womanhood and none of my "abilities" have been diminished. There were times in the past when I feared they had, but I know better now.

3. *Did you have reconstructive surgery?*

Ann: No. Although my doctor told me that I was a perfect candidate for reconstructive surgery, I thought that I had already asked enough of my body. It had been through the trauma and shock of a double mastectomy and I felt that I could go through life without breasts. I discussed this with Andy and he, too, felt that we both needed to confront the fact that my breasts were gone—a reality that sooner or later every woman who has had a mastectomy must deal with and accept. Neither of us felt we needed to have a reasonable facsimile. So I decided to wear my prosthesis on the outside of my body rather than going through surgeries to wear it on the inside. I believe it is every woman's personal decision. Whatever choice she makes is fine, and I will defend her right to make that choice.

Martha: No. My surgery was too drastic to even consider it. However, even if I had been a perfect candidate for reconstruction I wouldn't have wanted it.

In the past I had to have surgeries that were not optional. They were necessary to save my life. Enough is enough.

My own personal opinion is that reconstruction is just as "fake" as an external prosthesis. I would never have considered the "ordeal" (it would be for me) for one moment unless Bob had wanted me to do it. I would do anything for him. I know that there is a real danger of infection with reconstruction and it just wouldn't have been worth the risk.

But remember: This is my personal opinion. Each woman has to weigh the pros and cons and decide for herself, if she has the option.

4. What was it like taking chemotherapy?

Martha: A nightmare that wouldn't stop. Chemotherapy, by far, was the most devastating part of the ordeal. Losing my hair (everywhere) was emotionally debilitating, embarrassing, humiliating, but the nausea was so horrible I have no words to describe it.

There seemed to be no end to it; no relief from it. It would last from one treatment to the next. The doctor tried valiantly to relieve some of my suffering and misery; but with little effect. I took an antinausea compound until my battered body totally rebelled and side effects from that drug simulated a stroke with paralysis. Each time I entered the hospital for a treatment my veins were worse; they finally collapsed. The nurses (all experts in IV treatment) couldn't get the needles into them either for chemo or to administer glucose and vitamins since I couldn't take anything by mouth. After repeated attempts they succeeded in putting the IV in one arm only to have to move it hours later to another arm or my hand because the fluid infiltrated the tissue.

I could go on and on about other chemo side effects such as dry mouth, ulcerated esophagus, and dry skin, but the nausea was by far the worst. I was totally debilitated by it.

Ann: Nausea was the worst part of the entire ordeal. Some people can take chemo and not suffer serious side effects, but I'm not one of them. I had severe nausea, and on treatment days I would start throwing up five or six hours after the injections. Sometimes there would be bleeding from my battered stomach. This scared me until the doctors reassured me that I would be all right.

I experienced some hair loss, but not all of it. My hair did grow back thicker when the treatments stopped.

Sometimes I had a burning sensation up my back and in my groin area, and a feeling like hot fluid was running in my veins.

I could not eat or keep down any food, and often had a metallic taste in my mouth. Unfortunately, the antinausea drugs only made my nausea worse. I was offered cannabis (marijuana in pill form) because it sometimes has a calming effect on cancer patients. I refused, however, because I would rather know when I'm going to be sick than to be out of it on cannabis, and start throwing up in the living room instead of in the bathroom.

5. Can you still be sexy?

Ann: Yes. Why not? If all a person has is a good body they will soon discover that it is not enough to maintain an ongoing relationship. A good body might be enough for a sexual encounter, but it is not enough to maintain the intimate relationship that sustains a marriage. I believe that true sexiness comes from within.

Martha: Yes, I believe I'm still sexy. Like I said, I didn't lose *everything*. I just try to make what I do have even better—mentally as well as physically. Of course I continue to take pride in my appearance, including dress, personal hygiene, makeup, hairstyles, etc.

6. Can you still have a baby?

Ann: Yes, but people's circumstances vary and this is not true of all women who have had breast cancer. Sometimes a woman chooses not to have a baby, for fear of passing along to a daughter the higher risk of developing breast cancer. Each woman's case is unique, and decisions should be based on discussions with a doctor. There is only one thing I can't do and that is nurse a baby, but there are bottles!

Martha: I don't know. But at this point in my life I am not interested. I have two grown children and I feel very fulfilled in that area of my life. However, if a woman desires to have a child after breast cancer, I don't see why not. Of course, discuss it with your doctor.

7. How has having had breast cancer affected your career as an actress and singer?

Ann: The only thing I can't do is show cleavage. I never did any nude work, so I'm not missing out on that. I have found that—at last—my acting is now being taken more seriously than prior to my surgery.

(Ann has received three Emmy nominations and one Golden Globe award for best actress.)

My singing has been unaffected. If anything, song lyrics now take on more significance than ever before. I can even sing the blues, if I choose to. Torch songs and ballads have always been my specialty and now more than ever, they go over exceptionally well with audiences in my concerts and Atlantic City and Vegas shows.

> *8. Have you suffered any discrimination because you have had cancer?*

Ann: This is a legal bomb. Before an actor is hired for a project, he must pass a physical to certify that he will finish the picture. About all I can say is that I have been suspicious of some requests for additional medical reports or more comprehensive medical checkups as opposed to the routine checkup of listening to your heart, looking down your throat, and sending you off to work. But to date, all insurance companies have approved me for my film work. And I have never missed a day on the job for *any* reason.

Martha: I'm a housewife and don't work outside the home. I've never had an experience with discrimination in public or private of which I am aware.

> *9. What was the single most important lesson you learned?*

Ann: Early detection can save your life!

Martha: Improvement is something that always takes place in the future. With my future appearing to be limited, I discovered that change had to take place in the present.

So I borrowed that old cliché, "Never put off until tomorrow what you can do today." And I applied that to things both physical and spiritual. I learned that I wanted to improve the quality of my character now, and not later. I wanted to try to be a more caring, generous, unselfish, and kind person, not that I was a Lizzie Borden or a Simon Legree, but we can all improve.

> *10. What was it like the first time you appeared on stage after your surgery?*

Ann: It was at a benefit performance in Dallas on May fifth, 1985. I was cobilled with Bob Hope and even though it was less than a month since the surgery, I knew I would make that date. Nervous? You bet. Scared? Absolutely. I felt like a big chunk of my career was riding on this one performance. The predominate thought? How would the audience accept me?

There is no way I can describe the clash of emotions as I walked onstage in front of a live audience for the first time after my surgery. When I had gone back to work on "Alice," it was a controlled situation. If I needed it, I could get a second take. But that night, it was now or never. Success or failure.

It was time. My intro music was playing, I gathered my courage, and walked onto the stage singing. It was such an amazing sight, I had to quit singing. The audience, all in formal attire, was standing, and it seemed like a rock concert, a jumble of music and applause and cheering and whistling. I was overwhelmed. I remember thinking, "You're not going to cry." But I did. Then I tried to sing again, but the ovation was too loud and I couldn't hear enough of the music to know where I was. The audience realized the problem, I think, and the applause lessened, so my conductor (Nelson Kole) started again and this time I heard the music and we were off and running.

I didn't think about cancer or illness or anything like that throughout the rest of the evening; until my final number when I tried to raise my arm straight to the sky. It couldn't go that high because of the surgery, so I sort of twisted my body in a curve to make it appear I had extended it all the way. As I held the note, I was exhilarated. I remember thinking, "I have work to do, I know I'm not a hundred percent yet, but I will be." My arm had nearly made it straight up. For me this silly little dramatic act of extending an arm toward the sky revealed so much. As the audience applauded, my mind wandered back to the first time I tried to scratch behind my ear with my own hand and couldn't do it to as recently as a few minutes before when I had finger-wall-walked in my dressing room in anticipation of this performance.

But the big question had been answered the moment I stepped on the stage. There had been acceptance; even more than that, there had been love. The audience told me what I needed to know: "You're back," their applause said. "You are going to be given a chance to continue the work you love." This performance became both a turning point and a symbol. It proved that life goes on. In the future I discovered that the songs that received more applause before my surgery still received more applause afterward. Some jokes still got big laughs and that one joke that just didn't seem to go over, still fell flat on its face. The audience continued to judge me on talent, efforts, material, and performance.

But that night in Dallas put me back in control. It was my life and my future and that audience will always have a special spot in my heart.

11. *Did you have any problems with fluids in your arms? And how long did it take before you could raise your arms over your head?*

Ann: I had a little problem with fluid collecting in my arms since it no longer went through the lymph glands. I experienced soreness, slight pain, and some swelling. But I found that my exercises—raising my hands over my head and making and releasing fists—caused the fluid to circulate better.

It took about six to eight weeks before I was able to raise my arms over my head. It happened one day while I was gardening (with heavy gloves on as doctors advise against any cuts). A bougainvillea fell from up high and in self-defense, I put my hands up to catch it so that it wouldn't hit my face. It was a few seconds before I realized that my arms were over my head. I kept them up and ran to the rear of the house looking for Andy and yelling like crazy, "They're up, they're up!"

To help me achieve this goal, Andy used to play a game of stick 'em up. He'd pass me in the halls and point his finger at me like he had a pistol and say "Stick 'em up. Reach for the sky, baby face!" I'd have to put my arms up as high as I could and he would say, "Come on, you can go higher than that." I'd strain and try harder and then he'd say, "Okay, make your fists for the fluid," and I'd have to pump my fists fifty times. Only then would he let me pass into the next room. It was a pain if I was in a hurry, but it paid off. I have great use of my limbs and no more pain or swelling.

Martha: Yes, some fluid collected in my arms. I find that if I'm diligent in doing my exercises (holding my arms up and making a tight fist and releasing it), it takes care of the problem.

It took me a year before I could raise my left arm over my head. This is something I had to work on each day.

12. *Was there any history of breast cancer in your family and do you think a woman is at higher risk to get breast cancer if she has a blood relative who has had it?*

Ann: Yes, a very close relative had it some thirty years ago and is still alive and well now. Andy lost both his mother and sister to cancer. In fact, Dr. Michael Swift of the University of North Carolina at Chapel Hill has identified a gene that is directly tied to breast cancer. A woman who carries this gene has nearly seven times the risk of getting breast cancer. If a close relative has had breast cancer, you should be on guard and monitor your own situation very closely.

Martha: No. To my knowledge, there was absolutely no history of breast cancer or cancer at all in my family. I've probed my memory about this and have talked to older family members. None of them can remember a case of cancer, either.

13. *Did you or your doctor find your first lump?*

Ann: I did, during routine BSE (breast self-examination). It was a pea-sized lump on my left breast, very hard in substance, and it came and went with my menstrual cycle. It was difficult to find sometimes and easy at others.

Martha: I found lumps periodically. They were diagnosed as fibrocystic cysts, which are found in so many women that a debate is raging among doctors as to whether they are a "disease" or a "natural" condition. The doctors said that the only way to be a hundred percent sure was to perform a biopsy.*

I elected to have a regular mammogram and to have the lumps aspirated rather than go through surgery. It was more than a year later that one of the lumps could not be aspirated and it was discovered to be cancer.

14. Did the surgery hurt? Was there much pain?

Ann: Oddly enough, no. There was little pain. In fact, I felt great after the surgery; I got sick only when the precautionary chemotherapy treatments started. To me, that was the worst part.

Martha: Yes, of course. There is always some pain with surgery. The amount of pain varies from person to person. The biopsy was as painless as any surgery can be. The incision was so small—less than one-and-a-half inches—that it was held together with tape rather than stitches.

Compared to some other surgeries I've had (kidney and colon), the pain of a simple mastectomy or even a modified radical mastectomy is nominal because the surgeon does not cut into your body cavity.

15. Why didn't you have a lumpectomy instead of having both your breasts removed?

Ann: With all the publicity given lumpectomies, this is a question I'm asked frequently. There are certain conditions that must be present before a lumpectomy can be considered as the surgery of choice. There is also a certain amount of risk (although some will argue with me on this opinion) with a lumpectomy. Will the cancer recur in the rest of the breast? You need to consider the fact that it is the same fatty tissue where the first cancer grew. Other factors include the size of the tumor and the age of the woman. Still another is the type of cancer. And, patient history is likely to place certain women in a higher-risk category.

---

*Fibrocystic breast tissue is not necessarily cancerous, nor does having it make a woman an automatic candidate for developing breast cancer. Doctors and pathologists use mammograms, sonograms, and biopsies to look for "atypical" cells, which can develop in any type of breast tissue, fibrocystic or not. Mammograms are a valuable diagnostic tool in that they can identify a tumor as much as three to five years before such a tumor could be identified by breast self-examination. It is for this reason that the American Cancer Society recommends that all women over age thirty-five get a baseline mammogram. Mammograms, however, are not one hundred percent accurate or conclusive and therefore biopsies are often recommended to remove any doubt. A biopsy is what doctors recommended in Martha's case.

It takes examination, investigation, and much deliberation to determine which type of surgery is best for an individual.

It is an extremely personal decision based on individual factors. Martha and I checked all of the alternatives and then had the surgery that was best for each of us. All surgery is aimed at one goal, *life,* so whatever gives you the best shot at life is the best surgery for you.

Martha: I did not have a lumpectomy because at the time of the biopsy, the cancer was so widespread a mastectomy couldn't even be performed. I had to undergo chemotherapy and radiation with the hope that the cancer would be reduced to the point where a mastectomy could be performed. I was *hoping and praying* for the chance to have a mastectomy. That puts a new twist on it, doesn't it?

Later, when the second breast started showing signs of fibrocystic disease, I elected to have a simple mastectomy. I didn't want to keep going into the hospital for biopsies or be concerned that cancer would recur in that breast.

16. *Do you think that male surgeons are telling women that the surgery of choice is the complete removal of the breast(s) when they know that this is an aggressive measure and that a lumpectomy would serve the patient just as well?*

Ann: I have heard this type of question many times and in my experience, my male surgeon could not have been more compassionate and kind. He had tears in his eyes when he told me what type of surgery he thought I should have to save my life. He said, "If you were my sister, Ann, I would advise this surgery and the only thing that can justify it is that I want to save your life."

Martha: This question strikes a nerve with me.

No. I do *not* think surgeons are telling women that the surgery of choice is the complete removal of the breast(s) when they know that this is an aggressive measure and that a lumpectomy would serve the patient just as well.

These dedicated professionals are trying to save our lives. I don't believe they can be sure that a lumpectomy will do that, if cancer is definitely present. There might be a few unscrupulous and uncaring doctors who would whack away unnecessarily, just to make a few extra dollars, but I believe they are very few.

Vanity is the name of the game here and if you would rather gamble with your life than lose your breast or breasts, that is your decision, but know the facts and don't be quick to criticize and condemn doctors. When I elected to lose my breasts, I knew it would be at great personal loss. I had voluptuous breasts and often friends called me Martha Mae or MM, as in Mae West and Marilyn Monroe. Also remember that your decision will affect those who love you and are close to you.

All I know is that on the day of my biopsy, I wouldn't have given two cents for my chances of seeing my son, then a freshman, graduate from dental school. He's now graduated and I am oh-so-glad to be alive.

17. *Did you gain weight after your surgery or while on chemotherapy?*

Ann: Yes, and how! This happened for a number of reasons. First, I was not as active right away as I was before. My husband was stuffing me with every kind of food known to mankind to make sure I got plenty of nutrients. I was ready and willing to get *fat*. We all associate extreme skinniness with cancer so I think it is a normal reaction to eat a lot to put weight on your bones.

The other reason for weight gain was that my "chemo cocktail" contained one drug that bloated me until my face (and other parts of my body) started looking like a balloon.

Finally one night at dinner, almost a year after my chemo treatments were over, Andy looked up and said, "Hey, babe, you're eating like you're going to the electric chair in the morning!" He was right. I was almost keeping up with him.

It was about this time that we were approached to tell the Ann Jillian story, so the next morning I asked Andy if our producer had said anything about my weight. He had told Andy that I was too fat and had to take some weight off to make the movie's early scenes. That did it. We called our friend Luretta. She set up a workout and diet schedule.

It was strict but it did the job. I worked out five days a week, two to three hours a day. I ate—and still eat—only the stuff that's good for me (not sweets) and I seldom eat after six P.M. I drink tea or liquids.

(I must backtrack a bit. You see, I had done all this before with Luretta's help, and had kept on the program for a month. I gained one pound! Figure that out! I got disgusted and quit, just like many other women. My doctor said it was common, that the fat cells were just not ready to break down because of chemotherapy, etc. This was some six months after my chemo treatment was finished.)

But the second time was the charm. At the end of a year, the weight started to come off. I took it off slowly as I was going for strength as well as a svelte figure. I think any sudden shock to our bodies is not good for us so I do not advise quick weight loss. Do it gradually and easily, while building strength and eating the right foods for proper nutrition.

Pick *your* time to get going, just don't let it go too long or get too far out of hand. Adding a lot of fatty tissue to our bodies is not good. In addition to making more places for cancer to go, we increase our potential for heart problems and high blood pressure.

Try to eat right. Make it good foods right from the start of your
new life and don't let your body take on too much weight. Common
sense and guidance from your doctors will tell you when it is time to
hit the diet and exercise trail.

Martha: Not while on chemotherapy. I was so sick from nausea
that I lost thirty pounds. But since the treatments ended, I have gained
a whopping eighty pounds. I guess I was so glad to be able to eat
again that I ate everything in sight. It was so good to have an appetite
and feel good. Now I'm trying desperately to undo what I have done.
I've lost only a couple of pounds, but at least I've stopped gaining.

18. What type of diet do you recommend?

Ann: A commonsense diet. I used to try every fad or quick
weight-loss diet that came out. I even harbor some suspicion that
perhaps some of the junk food I was eating was part of the reason
I developed breast cancer. There is so much we don't know about
new products and fad diets that by the time the patent pending is
finalized, we might discover that something in the diet was dangerous
and had already done its damage to those who tried it.

The diet of choice of most people recovering from cancer (or
trying to prevent cancer) is simple: whole grains, fruits, and vegetables, while taking care to eat everything in moderation. Salt-cured,
smoked, and charcoal-broiled foods contain carcinogens that can be
dangerous. (I rarely have a broiled steak, maybe three per year.)

Be moderate when it comes to alcoholic beverages. I might have
a glass of wine or a gulp of beer a few times a year. I can do without
alcohol.

In an area where there are so many varied points of view, one
fact keeps popping up: experts in the field seem to agree that the
evidence linking breast cancer to high-fat diets is particularly strong.

Martha: A good, commonsense diet that places an emphasis on
ACS guidelines: Eat lots of fruit, nuts, vegetables, whole grains, lean
poultry and fish, occasional veal and very little red meat. Eat only
low-fat or nonfat dairy products. No fried foods unless they're stir-
fried vegetables. In general, consume as few fats as possible and eat
many of your fruits and vegetables raw if you can.

I had only a minimal interest in nutrition in high school. Like
most teenagers I attended home economics class, but the teacher's
efforts were mostly wasted on our inattentive group. "Who needs to
know this?" I reasoned, before teasing with my friends: "I'm going to
have a maid to do all my cooking." After I married and started to rear
children, I learned *I* needed to know it and became an avid reader
on the subject.

Since my illness I've been even more interested in nutrition in
light of the ACS suggestion that a proper diet possibly can act as a

deterrent to cancer. And with Bob a diabetic, proper nutrition is a necessity in our home.

I've developed a salad and a stew that are among Bob's favorites. We try to eat the chef's salad at least once a day. You might like to try it.

CHEF SALAD

1 cup fresh spinach
1 cup lettuce
2 medium tomatoes, cut, chopped, or sliced
1 stalk celery, chopped
2 green onions, washed and chopped (optional)
½ bell pepper, chopped
½ cucumber, chopped
½ cup broccoli flowerlets
½ cup cauliflower
½ cup sliced turkey (or chicken) breast
24 2-inch cheese strips (lo-fat)
1 boiled egg, sliced

Combine vegetables in large salad bowl and arrange sliced meat, cheese, and egg on top. Add your favorite low-calorie dressing. Serves two.

In my family, a hot steamy stew is a big favorite so I try to serve it once a week. It makes a complete meal, so you don't have to prepare any other dishes, unless you add a fresh tossed salad.

STEWART'S STEW

1 pound carrots
4 medium potatoes
2 medium onions
4 cloves garlic (good for your blood pressure)
3 stalks celery
3 medium zucchini

¼ *medium cabbage head*
 1 *14½-ounce can tomatoes*
 2 *6-ounce cans tomato sauce*
 ½ *teaspoon salt (optional)*
 ½ *teaspoon black pepper*
 1 *pound beef or chicken or turkey (very lean ground beef
     must be browned, drained, and blotted of all grease);
     chicken or turkey should be cut in chunks.*

Wash and scrub all vegetables. *Do not peel them.* Cut into bite-size pieces. Cook carrots in two quarts water for ½ hour over medium heat. Add remaining ingredients and cook just until vegetables are tender. *Do not overcook!* (You'll lose vitamins and nutrients.)

Experiment with this basic dish. You can omit any of the vegetables (everyone likes some vegetables better than others) or add your favorites such as frozen corn or green beans when the stew is almost done.

19. *Did you have fibrocystic breasts before you discovered you had
     breast cancer?*

Ann: Yes, I did. That accounts for the three-month period that my doctor had me "watching" the small lump and didn't do a biopsy right away. I would advise getting a biopsy quickly in cases like mine. I would not have minded a slight scar on my breast from the procedure.

Martha: Yes. This was explained in Question 13.

20. *Did you find that your doctors took enough time to explain
     everything to you when you discovered you had cancer and had
     so much to decide?*

Ann: Yes! I often hear horror stories of women whose doctors did not spend much time with them and who, just a few minutes after dropping a bombshell, would turn and walk away to treat another patient just as the woman's questions were beginning to tumble out. All I say every time I hear this is: You have the wrong doctor!

If your doctor leaves you in the dark, then find another one. Get to the expert in the field who will give you the time and the information you need to make good, solid decisions. Time is money with medical professionals, and none of us has a right to waste their time and prevent them from helping others and earning their living, so, after the initial shock, prepare for each session. Write down your questions. Be prepared so you can get the maximum amount of information in the briefest amount of time. A husband or family member can be a big help here. I was very nervous and had a lot on my mind and really needed someone to remember the doctor's answers and tell me what was said at a later time. We should all try and have our crying time prior to our visit with the doctor. Let's use the doctor for medical advice. Let's use our hubby or a dear friend for emotional comfort.

Martha: I don't know. The news was so devastating I couldn't hear all the details at the time because my mind was so clogged with thoughts. Bob did most of the talking with the doctors and he and I discussed it later at home.

When it was time for surgery, the doctors explained our options in detail, and allowed us to participate in my treatment.

21. *Did you find that you had to rethink your clothes styles after your surgery?*

Ann: Yes. I very much had to rethink what I would wear. Most of my gowns that used to reveal cleavage had to go, but I did save a few by finding a good seamstress. By making some very practical design changes, I improved upon some of my favorites. Don't go tossing out all your clothing too quickly. Many things can be saved with a stitch here or there. (Of course, you may just want to baby yourself and get some good shopping in as most women love to do, and if you can afford it, *do it!*)

I certainly was *not* ready to buy a black dress and sit in a corner. After all, my occupation would not allow that and neither would I. I love clothes and I know I'm not alone here. I tried to keep many things I liked—such as bras—and had them equipped to hold my prosthesis. This way I felt a bit less change right away.

One of my favorites is a black lace, low-cut gown. After surgery, it was too low, so I visited a dressmaker who designed a new front. The black lace was extended up my chest to the neck. She put in a flesh-color backing that made it "appear" that I had on a low-cut gown when seen through the black lace.

A good imagination and someone handy with a needle will save many of your favorites.

I even took some of my favorite swimsuits in to be remodeled so I could wear them in my home pool with close friends and family. The weight of the prosthesis kept pulling the tops of the suit forward, so I had the seamstress put in stronger neck and shoulder straps to keep the suit up.

Martha: I sewed stretch fabric into my bras and was able to save most of them. I don't know if it's all in my mind or what, but I felt uncomfortable in prosthesis bras, although I tried to wear them for months after my first surgery. Sometimes I dress up the top of a blouse with a scarf or a lace collar. And there is that old standby, the brooch, if the blouse or dress doesn't button high enough.

22. *Did you find that your bout with breast cancer brought you closer to God?*

Ann: I always felt close to God, but, yes, the ordeal brought me much closer to my faith. I often give credit to this faith for having played such an all-important role in my recovery and in my ability to go on with life in a very positive manner.

Martha: No. I've always felt close to God. I have always been a religious person and looked forward to life after death. To me, this means that I must try to live a life here on earth that I feel will please God. The bout with breast cancer has just made this meeting with God seem closer at hand. This makes me want to try harder right *now* to be the best person I can be. I touched on some of this in Question 9.

23. *How do you handle the "recurrence" worry that many who have had cancer have to live with?*

Ann: In addition to the Stewarts' twenty-five-year plan, which we borrowed and upped to fifty years—and without sounding like a broken record—it is my faith. After you do all that you can do medically you must find a way to lessen the pressure of this recurrence worry that we all share. For me it was faith. I remain resigned to His will. View this as a time to "reaffirm" your "good health" as opposed to trying to discover if cancer has reappeared or not.

Martha: The best way I handle the "recurrence" worry is to try not to think about it. When it enters my mind, I try to think about pleasant things—have some mind control. If I didn't, it would drive me crazy. It would be very easy to dwell on this and fall into deep depression—even despondency. I have to fight it every day!

24. *Did you ever consider giving up? Stopping your surgery? Stopping your chemotherapy?*

Ann: I never considered giving up on living! This is not and never has been in my makeup. But I did consider giving up on chemo treatments. I hated them so much and was so fearful of their effect on me that I prayed they would be over soon. In fact, out of a voluntary six-month treatment plan, I completed four and a half months and did in fact stop then. I was taking the chemo as added, aggressive insurance.

Had I really *needed* to take the chemotherapy, I would have kept up until I got through the prescription. But I know how every person must feel who may be suffering bad side effects.

Chemotherapy is an individual thing. It's like weight loss or size—some of us never get fat and some of us look at food and we move up a dress size! Although it was difficult for me, others have a lesser or greater degree of trouble with it.

Life was always my goal, no matter what I had to do.

Martha: Not really. During chemotherapy there were fleeting thoughts such as: "This is not worth it" or "I can't take it any longer," but all the while I knew it would be worth it (if it worked) and that I probably could take it; and I did. That is, almost.

My oncologist had to stop the chemo by mouth about three weeks early because I was getting progressively weaker, but I had already had the "big guns" as he calls them—three times.

Life was what it was all about; and I had too many things yet to do.

25. *What did your husband do that was the most helpful during the treatment/recovery phase?*

Ann: He prayed with me and he kept my spirits up. He never let me feel alienated or hopeless because there was always a plan "B" or a plan "C," right on through "Z," and although it never happened, I always had a feeling that if none of those worked, he would have developed more plans that always featured H-O-P-E. He always made me feel secure. I never felt that if what was being used didn't work, then I was a goner. I always knew he had some other bullet to fire.

After he got over the initial shock of breast cancer, Andy became a constant source of good humor for me. Humor made me feel less self-conscious and brought my own good sense of humor out even more.

I didn't have to worry about my treatment because he checked and double-checked all the information that was coming at me so fast. He was constantly on the telephone to the doctors, meticulously writing down exactly what they said in his journal and keeping a list of alternatives (Plan A or B or C). He could explain so much in layman's terms after he read everything he could get his hands on about breast cancer. Andy, in fact, is a very knowledgeable person about breast cancer and I still lean on him today for correct information that I may need before speaking to groups.

I've saved the best until last, because he did something very special after everything was over and done with, and I challenge other men to do the same.

Andy has given me "cancer-free days." Those are days on which I do not have to hear the word even once or speak to anyone about their cancer or do a show or whatever. He usually plans the day so I'm in my favorite place: our backyard where I can work with my flowers or enjoy the serenity of the well-kept lawn. He also has my family over for the day. I'm not allowed to go to the telephone that day if it's about cancer. He knows that I want to help others, but he also knows that I need a little "clearing out time" to give the old noodle a rest.

If you haven't done this for your wife, I urge you to do so.

Martha: The best thing for me was knowing that he was always there and that he loved me. Knowing that he would do anything within his power to help me; to help me get well; to survive; to feel better.

I love the words to the song "Lean on Me." The lyrics have a special meaning to me when the performer sings, "Lean on me, when you're not strong" because that's exactly what I did. I leaned on him because I wasn't strong—I was weak and sick. Physically he was strong, emotionally he was shaken, but still strong. I was afraid. I did not want to be alone for one moment. Of course, I had to be. Bob had to go to work to earn our living; but I knew that just as soon as he could, he would be home with me. In the meantime, he would call often to check on me. In the hospital he would order a rollaway bed and stay with me. A hospital room can be so lonely in the middle of the night. Just looking over at him asleep was comforting. Of course, hospitals are not my idea of a fun place to be, but if Bob had to be in one I would be by his side every minute I could—and he was there by mine.

These are the biggies Bob did. There are thousands of little things, far too many to mention.

26. *In retrospect, what did your husband do that was more of a hindrance than a help.*

Ann: As much as I love those big ol' puppy dog eyes, it always seemed like they had a "death look" in them right after my diagnosis. It got to the point that I had to tell him, "Don't look at me with those sad eyes. Please let me see life in your eyes."

I am proud to say that in spite of losing his mother and sister to cancer, very early on in my battle he learned there *can* be life and developed a positive outlook.

He was often too protective before he finally learned I wouldn't break.

He was too quick to read too much into my reactions to situations and didn't trust my real ability to adjust, often reading things into and beyond my answers or meanings.

His good intentions sometimes hampered me on the days of chemotherapy treatment. At one point he thought I was talking myself into being nauseous, but soon learned better when he tried so many ways to keep me from thinking about it, only to fail when everything came up, anyway.

He insisted that my parents be involved in my care on chemo nights. They would all gather around and take turns taking me to the bathroom to be sick. Andy insisted that we all handle this like a good family and their presence would demonstrate that they all loved me. I never thought it was necessary and I thought it was a strain on my elderly parents and my brother, who is a very quiet individual. Andy would have been enough to care for me on those long nights.

So, men, respect your wives' wishes regarding family and her care and do it "her way." I found having my family there just created more stress for me.

Martha: There are a couple of things that I wish hadn't happened.

He was too diligent with my exercises when I came home after the first surgery. Now I have trouble getting him away from the computer and out the door to go to the spa, take a walk, or work around the house.

Sometimes his attempt at "black humor" turned me off. He used to tell me I had a positive attitude because I was positive I was going to die. That wasn't too funny.

When it comes to handling illness, he had had a lot of practice before I was diagnosed as having cancer, so he already knew the ropes and that left less room for mistakes.

There are other things, but, as Bob says, "If you've been married to someone for more than twenty-five years, you could pick them to pieces because no one knows their faults better than you do."

I prefer to dwell on the good.

27. *What advice would you have for a woman to make this period easier on her husband and help him to help her?*

Ann: Be truthful, for starters. Don't let him become a Johnny-come-lately in the battle. I did that to Andy and it was so nice when he became involved. And being involved is what he wanted; it made it easier on him.

After a bit you might discover that you're laying everything on your husband, so pick someone else—a member of your family—and give your husband a break. Sometimes it gets rough for him. It's tough watching someone you love suffer.

Honesty. Honesty. Honesty. That's your watchword. And you want to watch for his emotional limits. He might need you as much as you need him during these times. Let him have a good cry every once in a while. You might even encourage him to cry with you.

Sometimes the two of you crying together—sort of a shared mourning—can work wonders on your outlook the next day.

Tell him exactly what you need and what you want, and watch his emotional reaction to judge if it's too much for him.

Don't forget to put your arms around your guy every once in a while. Let him know you care for him and what a great job he's doing for you.

Martha: Let him know that you realize he is suffering also. Sure, you're the one who has the actual physical disease and all that goes with it: surgery, pain, chemotherapy, nausea, radiation burns—the list is long. But you both suffer mental anguish and emotional upheaval. You fear death—him losing you and you losing him. It's agony for him to stand by and see you suffer and not be able to do it for you or lessen the pain or nausea.

Communicate with him. Discuss all things openly so he will know that you feel for him as well as his hurting for you. That won't take it away, but you both will know that each is thinking of the other.

Be cooperative. Take your medicine, try to eat, try not to complain. This is difficult at times, but always try to consider his feelings and what will be the easiest way for him to do things, even if that's not the way you would cook this or clean that.

And, most important, don't forget to tell him that you love him.

28. *What would you tell a man who has just learned that his wife has breast cancer?*

Ann: My advice to any man whose wife has just been diagnosed as having breast cancer is to "be there." It sounds simple, but there is such truth and wisdom in simplicity. Be there for everything that she needs or nothing, but "be there."

I know we've stressed the need to proceed with a normal life. If that means returning to your regular activities (for example, cards with the boys or a special fishing trip), that's okay, as long as you know, *without doubt,* that your wife wants you to go and can handle being alone or with someone else for that period of time.

Developing sensitivity for your wife's needs right now is very important. You will learn if you're being too protective or being too inattentive. Adjust accordingly.

Be honest with one another. No woman expects you to know all the answers or be a rock every inch of the way. Emotional upheaval is an obvious result of such traumatic news. But the stabilizing factor is the support you give one another. We don't expect you to be superhuman. We do, however, rely upon the supposition that when we said "I do" and exchanged "I love you's" and agreed to be "committed," we knew what the deeper meaning of those words were.

Be there.
Share.
Care.
Show love and stability of purpose.
Pray.
Then think positively—together.

Martha: Try to understand the paralyzing fear that strikes when you first hear the word cancer. Short of death, it's unlike any other word you'll ever hear. And after you understand that, then be her physical and spiritual strength.

I encourage you to explore the spiritual with her. I encourage you to develop a sensitivity to her moods, to her desire to live, to her fears of not only death but also of an unknown future.

Put her first, and do it willingly because if she ever needed it, she needs now to be the center of your universe. In being that, she will find a reservoir of strength that even you don't know exists.

Touch her constantly. Hold her hand, caress her arm, brush her hair—anything that brings you into physical contact. Talk to her, ask her opinions and share confidences.

Smile and laugh in spite of all the problems. Laughter is contagious. Laughter is healing. Laughter is fun and in the fun of laughter, she will discover that life continues.

And, finally, say the magic words: I love you. Say them over and over and over. You can never say them enough.

Glossary

Adjuvant chemotherapy: The use of anticancer drugs after surgery in patients whose cancers are most likely to recur.

Anemia: Condition in which the number of red blood cells is less than normal. Symptoms include shortness of breath, lack of energy, and fatigue.

Axilla: The armpit area, which contains lymph nodes and channels, blood vessels, muscles, and fat.

Benign tumor: A noncancerous growth that does not spread to other parts of the body.

Biopsy: The removal and microscopic examination of tissue for purposes of diagnosis.
Conventional surgical biopsy: Removal of a palpable lump or thickening by the surgeon.
Excisional biopsy: A biopsy that removes (excises) all of the questionable tissue.
Incisional biopsy: A procedure in which the surgeon cuts into (incises) a suspicious area and removes a small sample.
Needle localization biopsy: A special biopsy technique used when the breast abnormality cannot be felt with the fingers and appears only through mammography. Before biopsy, the radiologist marks the suspicious area with needle(s) and often dye. The surgeon then locates and removes the marked area of tissue, and the biopsy specimen is X-rayed to be sure all the suspicious area has been removed.

BSE or breast self-examination: Monthly examination of the breast by the woman herself. (Warning signs of breast cancer can include lumps; clear, milky, or bloody discharge from the nipple; retraction of the nipple; scaly skin around the nipple; changes in skin color or texture; dimpled or "orange-peel" skin; swelling, redness, or heat in the breast; enlargement of the lymph node under the arm.)

Cancer: A general term for more than a hundred diseases characterized by abnormal and uncontrolled growth of cells. The resulting mass, or tumor, can invade and destroy surrounding normal tissues. Cancer cells from the tumor can spread through the blood or lymph (the clear fluid that bathes body cells) to start new cancers in other parts of the body.

Chemotherapy: Treatment with anticancer drugs.

Combination chemotherapy: The use of two or three anticancer medications to treat an individual cancer patient.

Combined modality treatment: The use of anticancer drugs in combination with surgery or radiation.

Cyst: A fluid-filled mass that is usually harmless and can be removed by aspiration or surgery.

Fibrocystic disease: Chronic cystic mastitis, fibroadenosis, mastodynia, mammary dysplasia, benign breast changes. A general term for a number of noncancerous breast conditions usually involving lumpiness and/or pain in the fibrous tissue of the breast with the formation of cysts or, more broadly, for any benign breast change.

Intravenous (IV): Within or into a vein.

Invasive breast cancer: Disease in which breast cancer cells have penetrated (invaded) surrounding breast tissue.

Malignant tumor: A growth of cancer cells.

Metastases: Cancer growths that started from cancer cells from another part of the body.

Lump: Any kind of mass in the breast or elsewhere in the body.

Lymph nodes: Bean-shaped structures scattered along the vessels of the lymph system through which tissue fluid normally drains. The node traps harmful organisms so that they don't enter the body's circulatory system. Breast examination includes a check of the lymph nodes in the armpit area for any swelling.

Lymph system: It removes wastes from body tissues and carries fluids to help the body fight infection.

Lumpectomy: Removal of a lump and a small amount of surrounding breast tissue. Currently used as an option for some small breast cancers.

Malignancy: Cells that will continue to grow geometrically and are considered cancerous.

Mammography: X-ray examination of the breast that often detects breast changes (including carcinoma *in situ* and invasive breast cancer) before they can be felt with the fingers. Mammography produces a black-and-white film called a *mammogram.*
   Xeromammography: A variation on a mammogram that uses a recording technique to produce a blue-and-white X-ray picture on special paper.
   Sonogram: The breast is submerged in water and a sound wave passes through it, providing a detailed look at the interior of the breast.

Mastectomy: The surgical removal of all or part of the breast and sometimes adjoining structures, usually done for breast cancer.

Menopause: The time of a woman's life when her menstrual period stops, sometimes called "change of life." This sometimes occurs with chemotherapy treatment and can be temporary or permanent.

Needle aspiration: A diagnostic technique in which a thin hypodermic needle is inserted into a lump that may be fluid-filled, and any fluid is withdrawn into the syringe. If the lump is a cyst, it collapses. Any suspicious fluid can be sent to the cytology laboratory for examination. Sometimes a special needle or a different technique is used to withdraw a tiny piece of tissue or several cells from a solid lump for biopsy.

Noninvasive: Also called breast carcinoma *in situ.* A breast change in which highly atypical cells are localized, that is, they may be pressing against adjoining breast tissue but they have not penetrated (invaded) it nor spread (metastasized) beyond the breast. Doctors differ about whether this condition marks the last stage of benign change or the first stage of breast cancer.

Oncologist: A doctor specializing in the treatment of cancer. He or she may further specialize in medicine, radiation, or surgery, but always in relation to cancer.

Palpation: Feeling the breast with the hands for any abnormality.

Pathology: The examination of tissues and body fluids to determine whether malignant cells are present and to ascertain the type of cells.

Pathologist: A doctor with special training in diagnosing disease from a sample of tissue.

Prognosis: The projected future course of the illness.

Prosthesis: A manufactured device to fill out a woman's figure once she has had a mastectomy. They come in all textures, sizes, shapes, and colors. Mostly they are constructed to a standard, but some prostheses are made to fit the individual.

Radiation therapy: Treatment using high-energy radiation from X-ray machines, cobalt, radium, or other sources.

Radiologist: A doctor with special training in diagnosing disease by studying X-ray negatives.

Reconstruction: The rebuilding, or restructuring, of the breast area following mastectomy. Sometimes performed at the time of mastectomy, but more often performed at a later date. There are various types of reconstruction, depending on the surgical procedure and the desires of the patient.

Recurrence: Reappearance of cancer at the same site (local), near the first site (regional), or in other areas of the body (metastases).

Remission: When cancer can no longer be found to be present but cannot be determined as cured.

Scan: A picture of a particular part of the body, such as brain, liver, or bones, produced by counting the radiation caused by radioactive substances injected to that part. A CAT scan gives a detailed picture of a cross-section of the body.

Side effects: Reactions to drugs that are usually temporary and reversible. They don't relate to drug effectiveness.

Tumor: A swelling or enlargement due to abnormal overgrowth of tissue. It can be cancerous or noncancerous.

Selected Reading

American Cancer Society, Arthur I. Holeb, et al, eds. *The American Cancer Society's Complete Book of Cancer: Prevention, Detection, Diagnosis, Treatment, Cure.* New York: Doubleday, 1986.

ACS. Anne Lindsey in consultation with Diane J. Fink, M.D. *The American Cancer Society Cookbook.* New York: Hearst Books, 1988. More than 200 recipes following nutritional guidelines to reduce cancer risk.

ACS. *Eating Smart.* 87-250M-No. 2042-LE. 1987. Guide for sensible food choices that follow American Cancer Society nutrition guidelines.

ACS. *Cancer Facts & Figures—1988.* 88-500M-No. 5008-LE. 1988 (Updated yearly). A statistical examination of all types of cancer in the 50 United States and Puerto Rico.

ACS. *Taking Control: 10 Steps to a Healthier Life and Reduced Cancer Risk.* 85-5MM-Rev. 5/87-No. 2019.05. 1987. Helpful hints to reduce risk of cancer.

ACS. *Talking With Your Doctor.* 87-10m-No. 4638PS. 1987. Helpful hints on communication with the doctors treating a cancer patient.

ACS. *Finding a Lump in Your Breast.* 83-200M-Rev. 1/84-No. 4586-PS. 1983. Overview of treatment from diagnosis through chemotherapy.

ACS. *What Is Known . . . What Is Suspected . . . What Is Myth: About Cancer Risk Factors.* 81-50M-Rev. 3/87-No. 2651-LE. 1987. A chart defining known cancer risk factors.

ACS. *Mammography: Saving More Lives.* 1/87 Code 510. 1987. Description of mammography as method to detect breast cancer early.

ACS. *Listen With Your Heart: Talking With the Cancer Patient.* 78-100M-Rev. 3/86-No. 4557-PS. 1983. Simple rules and etiquette to follow when talking to a cancer patient.

ACS. *The Proof Is in the Living.* 83-200M-No. 2620-LE. 1983. Brief discussion of alternate treatments.

ACS. *The Hopeful Side of Cancer.* 81-300M-Rev. 11/86-No. 2012-LE. 1981. Offers several success stories, plus provides guidelines to maintain vigilance against cancer.

ACS. *Cancer Word Book.* 85-(100M)-No. 2097-LE. 1985. Definitions of words, plus blank pages to add your own notes.

ACS. *Reach to Recovery.* 82-100M-4601-PS. 1982. Self-help group whose members visit mastectomy patients in the hospital.

ACS. *Cancer: Your Job, Insurance, and the Law.* 84-100M-4585-PS. 1984. Brief discussion of a cancer patient's legal rights.

ACS. Texas Division Inc. *Head Dressing: Options With Wigs and Wraps.* 10/86 Code 1076. 1986. Beautifully illustrated brochure of head wraps using a 32- to 36-inch scarf or cloth square. Available only in Texas.

U.S. Department of Health and Human Services, National Institutes of Health. *Radiation Therapy: A Treatment for Early Stage Breast Cancer.* NIH Publication No. 84-659. 1984. Detailed booklet explaining procedures, treatment and side effects.

NIH. Mastectomy: A Treatment for Breast Cancer. NIH Publication No. 87-658. 1987. Describes types of surgery and methods of recovery following surgery.

NIH. *Diet, Nutrition & Cancer Prevention: A Guide to Food Choices.* NIH No. 87-2878. 1987. Nutritional guide with sample menus.

NIH. *Chemotherapy and You: A Guide to Self-Help During Treatment.* NIH Publication No. 86-1136. 1986. Booklet which discusses chemical treatment, side effects and their control, as well as an appendix explaining the most common chemotherapy drugs. Also provides blank pages for notes.

NIH. *After Breast Cancer: A Guide to Followup Care.* NIH Publication No. 85-2400. 1985. Guidelines to follow after surgery.

NIH. *Taking Time: Support for People With Cancer and the People Who Care About Them.* NIH Publication No. 83-2059. 1983. This is a 58-page booklet that details the emotional problems facing cancer patients and their friends and family.

NIH. *When Someone in Your Family Has Cancer.* NIH Publication No. 86-2685. 1985. Guidelines to help everyone in the family unit deal with cancer.

Resources

The Cancer Information Center
By telephone:
Toll-free: 1–800–4–CANCER
Alaska: 1–800–638–6070
Hawaii: Oahu, 524–1234 (neighbor islands call collect)

By letter:
Office of Cancer Communications
National Cancer Institute
Bethesda, Maryland 20892

By dialing the above numbers you will automatically be routed to your local Cancer Information Service. If there is no Cancer Information Service in your area, it will automatically connect you with the National Cancer Information Service lines in Rockville, Maryland. The telephone lines are open weekdays from 9 A.M. until 10 P.M. and on Saturday from 10 A.M. to 6 P.M. You can take comfort that there is an ACS unit within phone reach of everyone in the United States.

If you specifically request it, Cancer Information Service will access Physician Data Query (PDQ) on their computer and read the state-of-the-art information to you over the telephone along with any information on the current available protocols. They will mail print-outs of these to physicians and possibly to patients, if requested.

American Cancer Society
90 Park Avenue
New York, N.Y. 10016
1–212–599–8200

1–800–ACS–2345 — The Cancer Response System, a toll-free information service offering up-to-date information on treatment, detection, prevention, and local services available from the American Cancer Society.

Three distinct programs:

Reach to Recovery was developed to assist women who have either had a mastectomy or are about to undergo one. CanSurmount and I Can Cope are general programs to bring together volunteers, health professionals, and individuals with cancer and their families to provide general information and physical and emotional support. Check your nearest American Cancer Society for a local telephone number for these support groups.

Make Today Count
P.O. Box 222
Osage Beach, Mo. 65065
1-314-348-1619

As the name implies, the goal is to help all cancer patients—in whatever stage of the battle—to "live each day as fully and completely as possible."

Medicaid/Medicare
Health Financing Administration
Department of Health and Human Services
Washington, D.C. 20201
1-202-245-0312

The home office can provide you with the address and telephone number of your regional office.

United Way
701 North Fairfax
Alexandria, Va. 22314
1-703-836-7100

Assistance and referral to a variety of services can be obtained through the local United Way agency.

American Psychiatric Association
1700 18th Street, N.W.
Washington, D.C. 20009
1-202-232-7878

This national organization of psychiatric specialists will be able to put you in touch with a local group.

American Psychological Association
1200 17th Street, N.W.
Washington, D.C. 20036
1-202-833-7600

This national organization of psychologists will be able to put you in touch with a local group.

Index